THE AMERICAN PSYCHIATRIC ASSOCIATION
PRACTICE GUIDELINES FOR THE
Psychiatric Evaluation
of Adults

THIRD EDITION

APA Work Group on Psychiatric Evaluation

Joel J. Silverman, M.D., *Chair*
Marc Galanter, M.D.
Maga Jackson-Triche, M.D., M.S.H.S.
Douglas G. Jacobs, M.D.
James W. Lomax II, M.D.
Michelle B. Riba, M.D.
Lowell D. Tong, M.D.
Katherine E. Watkins, M.D., M.S.H.S.

Systematic Review Group

Laura J. Fochtmann, M.D., M.B.I.
Richard S. Rhoads, M.D.
Joel Yager, M.D.

APA Steering Committee on Practice Guidelines

Michael J. Vergare, M.D., *Chair*
James E. Nininger, M.D., *Vice-Chair*
Thomas J. Craig, M.D.
Deborah Cowley, M.D.
Nassir Ghaemi, M.D., M.P.H.
David A. Kahn, M.D.
John M. Oldham, M.D.
Carlos N. Pato, M.D., Ph.D.
Mary S. Sciutto, M.D.

Assembly Area Liaisons

Daniel J. Anzia, M.D., *Chair of Area Liaisons* (and Area IV)
John M. de Figueiredo, M.D. (Area I)
Marvin Koss, M.D. (Area II)
William M. Greenberg, M.D. (Area III)
John P.D. Shemo, M.D. (Area V)
Robert M. McCarron, D.O. (Area VI)
Jason W. Hunziker, M.D. (Area VII)

APA wishes to acknowledge the contributions of former APA staff to these guidelines: Robert Kunkle, M.A., Robert Plovnick, M.D., Sara Reid, M.A., Seung-Hee Hong, and William E. Narrow, M.D., M.P.H.

APA and the Work Group on Psychiatric Evaluation especially thank Laura J. Fochtmann, M.D., M.B.I, and Robert Kunkle, M.A., for their outstanding work and effort on developing these guidelines.

The executive summary for this practice guideline was published by *The American Journal of Psychiatry* in 2015 (doi: 10.1176/appi.ajp.2015.1720501).

For inquiries about permissions or licensing, please contact Permissions & Licensing, American Psychiatric Publishing, 1000 Wilson Boulevard, Suite 1825, Arlington, VA 22209-3901 or submit inquiries online at: http://www.appi.org/CustomerService/Pages/Permissions.aspx.

If you wish to buy 50 or more copies of the same title, please go to www.appi.org/specialdiscounts for more information.

Manufactured in the United States of America on acid-free paper
19   18   17   16   5   4   3   2
Third Edition

American Psychiatric Association
1000 Wilson Boulevard
Arlington, VA 22209-3901
www.psych.org

Library of Congress Cataloging-in-Publication Data
APA Work Group on Psychiatric Evaluation, author.
   The American Psychiatric Association practice guidelines for the psychiatric evaluation of adults / APA Work Group on Psychiatric Evaluation, Joel J. Silverman, chair, [and eleven others]. — Third edition.
      p. ; cm.
   Practice guidelines for the psychiatric evaluation of adults.
   Includes bibliographical references.
   ISBN 978-0-89042-465-0 (pbk. : alk. paper)
   I. Silverman, Joel J., contributor. II. American Psychiatric Association, publisher. III. Title. IV. Title: Practice guidelines for the psychiatric evaluation of adults.
   [DNLM: 1. Adult. 2. Mental Disorders—diagnosis—Practice Guideline. 3. Interview, Psychological—methods—Practice Guideline. WT 150]
   RC469
   616.89′075—dc23
                                                                                      2015022857

British Library Cataloguing in Publication Data
A CIP record is available from the British Library.

Contents

Practice Guidelines for the Psychiatric Evaluation of Adults, Third Edition 9

Executive Summary

Background and Development Process

These Practice Guidelines for the Psychiatric Evaluation of Adults mark a transition in the American Psychiatric Association's Practice Guidelines. Since the publication of the Institute of Medicine (2011) report, "Clinical Practice Guidelines We Can Trust," there has been an increasing focus on using clearly defined, transparent processes for rating the quality of evidence and the strength of the overall body of evidence in systematic reviews of the scientific literature. These guidelines were developed using a process intended to be consistent with the recommendations of the Institute of Medicine (2011), the Principles for the Development of Specialty Society Clinical Guidelines of the Council of Medical Specialty Societies (2012), and the requirements of the Agency for Healthcare Research and Quality (AHRQ) for inclusion of a guideline in the National Guideline Clearinghouse. Parameters used for the guidelines' systematic review are included with the full text of the guidelines; the development process is fully described in a document available on the APA Web site: http://www.psychiatry.org/File%20Library/Practice/APA-Guideline-Development-Process--updated-2011-.pdf. To supplement the expertise of members of the guideline work group, we used a "snowball" survey methodology to identify experts on psychiatric evaluation and solicit their input on aspects of the psychiatric evaluation that they saw as likely to improve specific patient outcomes (Yager et al. 2014). Results of this expert survey are included with the full text of the practice guideline.

Rating the Strength of Research Evidence and Recommendations

The new guideline recommendations are rated using GRADE (Grading of Recommendations Assessment, Development and Evaluation), an approach adopted by multiple professional organizations around the world to develop practice guideline recommendations (Guyatt et al. 2008, 2013). With the GRADE approach, the strength of a guideline statement reflects the level of confidence that potential benefits of an intervention outweigh the potential harms (Andrews et al. 2013). This level of confidence is informed by available evidence, which includes evidence from clinical trials as well as expert opinion and patient values and preferences. Evidence for the benefit of a particular intervention within a specific clinical context is identified through systematic review and is then balanced against the evidence for harms. In this regard, harms are broadly defined and might include direct and indirect costs of the intervention (including opportunity costs) as well as potential for adverse effects from the intervention. Whenever possible, we have followed the admonition to current guideline development groups to avoid using words such as "might" or "consider" in drafting these recommendations because they can be difficult for clinicians to interpret (Shiffman et al. 2005).

As described under "Guideline Development Process," each final rating is a consensus judgment of the authors of the guidelines and is endorsed by the APA Board of Trustees. A "recommendation" (denoted by the numeral 1 after the guideline statement) indicates confidence that the benefits of the intervention clearly outweigh harms. A "suggestion" (denoted by the numeral 2 after the guideline statement) indicates uncertainty (i.e., the balance of benefits and harms is difficult to judge, or either the benefits or the harms are unclear). Each guideline statement also has an associated rating for the "strength of supporting research evidence." Three ratings are used: high, moderate, or low (denoted by the letters *A*, *B* and *C*, respectively) and reflect the level of confidence that the evidence reflects a true effect based on consistency of findings across studies, directness of the effect on a specific health outcome, and precision of the estimate of effect and risk of bias in available studies (AHRQ 2014; Balshem et al. 2011; Guyatt et al. 2006).

It is well recognized that there are guideline topics and clinical circumstances for which high-quality evidence from clinical trials is not possible or is unethical to obtain (Council of Medical Specialty Societies 2012). For example, it would not be ethical to randomly assign only half of patients with depression to be asked about suicidal ideas. Many questions need to be asked as part of the assessment, and inquiring about a particular symptom or element of the history cannot be separated out for study as a discrete intervention. It would also be impossible to separate changes in outcome due to assessment from changes in outcomes due to ensuing treatment. Research on psychiatric assessment is also complicated by multiple confounding factors, such as the interaction between the clinician and the patient or the patient's unique circumstances and experiences. For these and other reasons, the vast majority of topics covered in these guidelines on psychiatric evaluation have relied on forms of evidence such as consensus opinions of experienced clinicians or indirect findings from observational studies rather than being based on research from randomized trials. The GRADE working group and guidelines developed by other professional organizations have noted that a strong recommendation may be appropriate even in the absence of research evidence when sensible alternatives do not exist (Andrews et al. 2013; Brito et al. 2013; Djulbegovic et al. 2009; Hazlehurst et al. 2013).

Goals and Scope of Guidelines for the Psychiatric Evaluation of Adults

Despite the difficulties in obtaining quantitative evidence from randomized trials for practice guidelines such as psychiatric evaluation, guidance to clinicians can still be beneficial in enhancing care to patients. Thus, in the context of an initial psychiatric evaluation, a major goal of these guidelines is to improve the identification of psychiatric signs and symptoms, psychiatric disorders (including substance use disorders), other medical conditions (that could affect the accuracy of a psychiatric diagnosis), and patients who are at increased risk for suicidal or aggressive behaviors. Additional goals relate to identifying factors that could influence the therapeutic alliance, enhance clinical decision making, enable safe and appropriate treatment planning, and promote better treatment outcomes. Finally, the psychiatric evaluation is the start of a dialog with patients about many factors, including diagnosis and treatment options. Further goals of these guidelines are to improve collaborative decision making between patients and clinicians about treatment-related decisions as well as to increase coordination of psychiatric treatment with other clinicians who may be involved in the patient's care.

Time Required to Complete a Psychiatric Evaluation

It is essential to note that these guidelines are not intended to be comprehensive in scope. Many critical aspects of the psychiatric evaluation are not addressed by these guidelines. For example, it is assumed that initial psychiatric or other medical assessments will need to identify the reason that the patient is presenting for evaluation. It is similarly important to understand the patient's background, relationships, life circumstances, strengths, and vulnerabilities.

Furthermore, depending on the context, recommended areas of inquiry may need to be postponed until later visits, and recommended questions will not always be indicated for a specific patient. The findings of the expert survey reiterate that experts vary in the extent to which particular elements of the initial psychiatric evaluation are assessed. This also highlights the importance of clinical judgment in tailoring the psychiatric evaluation to the unique circumstances of the patient and in determining which questions are most important to ask as part of an initial assessment.

Proper Use of Guidelines

The APA Practice Guidelines are not intended to serve or be construed as a "standard of medical care." Judgments concerning clinical care depend on the clinical circumstances and data available for an individual patient and are subject to change as scientific knowledge and technology advance and practice patterns evolve. These guideline statements were determined on the basis of the relative balance of potential benefits and harms of a specific assessment, intervention, or other approach to care. As such, it is not possible to draw conclusions about the effects of omitting a particular recommendation, either in general or for a specific patient. Furthermore, adherence to these guidelines will not ensure a successful outcome for every individual, nor should these guidelines be interpreted as including all proper methods of evaluation and care or excluding other acceptable methods of evaluation and care aimed at the same results. The ultimate recommendation regarding a particular assessment, clinical procedure, or treatment plan must be made by the psychiatrist in light of the psychiatric evaluation, other clinical data, and the diagnostic and treatment options available. Such recommendations should be made in collaboration with the patient and family, whenever possible, and incorporate the patient's personal and sociocultural preferences and values in order to enhance the therapeutic alliance, adherence to treatment, and treatment outcomes.

Organization of the Practice Guidelines for the Psychiatric Evaluation of Adults

As part of aligning the practice guidelines' development process with national standards, we have transitioned to a new guideline format. Each set of Practice Guidelines will consist of multiple discrete topics of relevance to an overall subject area. In the Practice Guidelines for the Psychiatric Evaluation of Adults, these topics consist of Review of Psychiatric Symptoms, Trauma History, and Psychiatric Treatment History; Substance Use Assessment; Assessment of Suicide Risk; Assessment of Risk for Aggressive Behaviors; Assessment of Cultural Factors; Assessment of Medical Health; Quantitative Assessment; Involvement of the Patient in Treatment Decision Making; and Documentation of the Psychiatric Evaluation. For each topic, guideline statements will be followed by a discussion of the rationale, potential benefits and harms, and approaches to implementing the guideline statements. This portion of the Practice Guidelines is expected have the greatest utility for clinicians. A second section of the Practice Guidelines provides a detailed review of the evidence for guideline statements in accord with national guideline development standards. This review of research evidence and data from the expert survey is followed by a discussion of quality measurement considerations, including their appropriateness for each topic.

Guideline Statements

The following represents a summary of the recommendations and suggestions compiled from all Practice Guidelines for the Psychiatric Evaluation of Adults, with some statements being a part of more than one of these guidelines. In the context of these guideline statements, it is important to note that assessment is not limited to direct examination of the patient. Rather, it is defined as "[t]he process of obtaining information about a patient through any of a variety of methods, including face-to-face interview, review of medical records, physical examination (by the psychiatrist, another physician, or a medically trained clinician), diagnostic testing, or history-taking from collateral sources." The evaluation may also require several meetings, with the patient, family, or others, before it can be completed. The amount of time spent depends on the complexity of the problem, the clinical setting, and the patient's ability and willingness to cooperate with the assessment.

This summary is organized according to common headings of an evaluation note. As noted above, the guidelines are not intended to be comprehensive, and many aspects of the psychiatric evaluation are not addressed by these recommendations and suggestions. Recommendations for the initial psychiatric evaluation of a patient appear in bold font, whereas suggestions appear in italic font. The strength of supporting research evidence for these recommendations and suggestions is given rating C (low) because of the difficulties in studying psychiatric assessment approaches in controlled studies as described above. References to the specific guideline in which the recommendation or suggestion is found are denoted by the following footnotes:

[1] Guideline I. Review of Psychiatric Symptoms, Trauma History, and Psychiatric Treatment History

[2] Guideline II. Substance Use Assessment

[3] Guideline III. Assessment of Suicide Risk

[4] Guideline IV. Assessment of Risk for Aggressive Behaviors

[5] Guideline V. Assessment of Cultural Factors

[6] Guideline VI. Assessment of Medical Health

[7] Guideline VII. Quantitative Assessment

[8] Guideline VIII. Involvement of the Patient in Treatment Decision Making

[9] Guideline IX. Documentation of the Psychiatric Evaluation

History of Present Illness

- **Reason that the patient is presenting for evaluation:**
  - **Psychiatric review of systems,[1] including anxiety symptoms and panic attacks[3]**
  - **Past or current sleep abnormalities, including sleep apnea[6]**
  - **Impulsivity[3,4]**

Psychiatric History

- **Past and current psychiatric diagnoses[1,3]**
- **Prior psychotic or aggressive ideas, including thoughts of physical or sexual aggression or homicide[4]**
- **Prior aggressive behaviors (e.g., homicide, domestic or workplace violence, other physically or sexually aggressive threats or acts)[4]**
- **Prior suicidal ideas, suicide plans, and suicide attempts, including attempts that were aborted or interrupted as well as the details of each attempt (e.g., context, method, damage, potential lethality, intent)[3]**
- **Prior intentional self-injury in which there was no suicide intent[3]**
- **History of psychiatric hospitalization and emergency department visits for psychiatric issues[1,3,4]**
- **Past psychiatric treatments (type, duration, and, where applicable, doses)[1]**
- **Response to past psychiatric treatments[1]**

- Adherence to past and current pharmacological and nonpharmacological psychiatric treatments[1]

Substance Use History

- Use of tobacco, alcohol, and other substances (e.g., marijuana, cocaine, heroin, hallucinogens) and any misuse of prescribed or over-the-counter medications or supplements[2]
- Current or recent substance use disorder or change in use of alcohol or other substances[3,4]

Medical History[6]

- Allergies or drug sensitivities
- All medications the patient is currently or recently taking and the side effects of these medications (i.e., both prescribed and nonprescribed medications, herbal and nutritional supplements, and vitamins)
- Whether or not the patient has an ongoing relationship with a primary care health professional
- Past or current medical illnesses and related hospitalizations
- Relevant past or current treatments, including surgeries, other procedures, or complementary and alternative medical treatments
- Past or current neurological or neurocognitive disorders or symptoms[4]
- Physical trauma, including head injuries
- Sexual and reproductive history
- *Cardiopulmonary status*
- *Past or current endocrinological disease*
- *Past or current infectious disease, including sexually transmitted diseases, HIV, tuberculosis, hepatitis C, and locally endemic infectious diseases such as Lyme disease*
- *Past or current symptoms or conditions associated with significant pain and discomfort*

Review of Systems[6]

- Psychiatric (if not already included with history of present illness)
- *Constitutional symptoms (e.g., fever, weight loss)*
- *Eyes*
- *Ears, nose, mouth, throat*
- *Cardiovascular*
- *Respiratory*
- *Gastrointestinal*
- *Genitourinary*
- *Musculoskeletal*
- *Integumentary (skin and/or breast)*
- *Neurological*
- *Endocrine*
- *Hematological/lymphatic*
- *Allergic/immunological*

Family History

- History of suicidal behaviors in biological relatives (for patients with current suicidal ideas)[3]
- History of violent behaviors in biological relatives (for patients with current aggressive ideas)[4]

Personal and Social History

- Presence of psychosocial stressors (e.g., financial, housing, legal, school/occupational or interpersonal/relationship problems; lack of social support; painful, disfiguring, or terminal medical illness)[3,4]
- Review of the patient's trauma history[1,3]
- Exposure to violence or aggressive behavior, including combat exposure or childhood abuse[4]
- Legal or disciplinary consequences of past aggressive behaviors[4]
- Cultural factors related to the patient's social environment[5]
- *Personal/cultural beliefs and cultural explanations of psychiatric illness*[5]
- Patient's need for an interpreter[5]

Examination, Including Mental Status Examination

- General appearance and nutritional status[6]
- *Height, weight, and body mass index (BMI)*[6]
- *Vital signs*[6]
- *Skin, including any stigmata of trauma, self-injury, or drug use*[6]
- Coordination and gait[6]
- Involuntary movements or abnormalities of motor tone[6]
- Sight and hearing[6]
- Speech, including fluency and articulation[6]
- Mood, level of anxiety, thought content and process, and perception and cognition[1,3]
- Hopelessness[3]
- Current suicidal ideas, suicide plans, and suicide intent, including active or passive thoughts of suicide or death[3]
  - If current suicidal ideas are present, assess
    - Patient's intended course of action if current symptoms worsen
    - Access to suicide methods including firearms
    - Patient's possible motivations for suicide (e.g., attention or reaction from others, revenge, shame, humiliation, delusional guilt, command hallucinations)
    - Reasons for living (e.g., sense of responsibility to children or others, religious beliefs)
    - Quality and strength of the therapeutic alliance
  - Current aggressive or psychotic ideas, including thoughts of physical or sexual aggression or homicide[3,4]
  - If current aggressive ideas are present, assess
    - Specific individuals or groups toward whom homicidal or aggressive ideas or behaviors have been directed in the past or at present
    - Impulsivity, including anger management issues
    - Access to firearms

Impression and Plan

- Documentation of an estimate of the patient's suicide risk, including factors influencing risk[3]
- Documentation of the rationale for treatment selection, including discussion of the specific factors that influenced the treatment choice[9]
- Asking the patient about treatment-related preferences[8]

- An explanation to the patient of the following: the differential diagnosis, risks of untreated illness, treatment options, and benefits and risks of treatment[8]
- Collaboration between the clinician and the patient about decisions pertinent to treatment[8]
- *Quantitative measures of symptoms, level of functioning, and quality of life*[7]
- *Documentation of an estimated risk of aggressive behavior (including homicide), including factors influencing risk*[4]
- *Documentation of the rationale for clinical tests*[9]

References

Agency for Healthcare Research and Quality: Methods Guide for Effectiveness and Comparative Effectiveness Reviews. AHRQ Publ No 10(14)-EHC063-EF. Rockville, MD, Agency for Healthcare Research and Quality. January 2014. Chapters available at: www.effectivehealthcare.ahrq.gov.

Andrews JC, Schünemann HJ, Oxman AD, et al: GRADE guidelines: 15. Going from evidence to recommendation-determinants of a recommendation's direction and strength. J Clin Epidemiol 66(7):726–735, 2013 23570745

Balshem H, Helfand M, Schünemann HJ, et al: GRADE guidelines: 3. Rating the quality of evidence. J Clin Epidemiol 64(4):401–406, 2011 21208779

Brito JP, Domecq JP, Murad MH, et al: The Endocrine Society guidelines: when the confidence cart goes before the evidence horse. J Clin Endocrinol Metab 98(8):3246–3252, 2013 23783104

Council of Medical Specialty Societies (CMSS): Principles for the Development of Specialty Society Clinical Guidelines. Chicago, IL, CMSS, 2012

Djulbegovic B, Trikalinos TA, Roback J, et al: Impact of quality of evidence on the strength of recommendations: an empirical study. BMC Health Serv Res 9:120, 2009 19622148

Guyatt G, Gutterman D, Baumann MH, et al: Grading strength of recommendations and quality of evidence in clinical guidelines: report from an american college of chest physicians task force. Chest 129(1):174–181, 2006 16424429

Guyatt GH, Oxman AD, Kunz R, et al; GRADE Working Group: Going from evidence to recommendations. BMJ 336(7652):1049–1051, 2008 18467413

Guyatt G, Eikelboom JW, Akl EA, et al: A guide to GRADE guidelines for the readers of JTH. J Thromb Haemost 11(8):1603–1608, 2013 23773710

Hazlehurst JM, Armstrong MJ, Sherlock M, et al: A comparative quality assessment of evidence-based clinical guidelines in endocrinology. Clin Endocrinol (Oxf) 78(2):183–190, 2013 22624723

Institute of Medicine (IOM): Clinical Practice Guidelines We Can Trust. Washington, DC, The National Academies Press, 2011

Shiffman RN, Dixon J, Brandt C, et al: The GuideLine Implementability Appraisal (GLIA): development of an instrument to identify obstacles to guideline implementation. BMC Med Inform Decis Mak 5:23, 2005 16048653

Yager J, Kunkle R, Fochtmann LJ, et al: Who's your expert? Use of an expert opinion survey to inform development of American Psychiatric Association practice guidelines. Acad Psychiatry 38(3):376–382, 2014 24493361

PRACTICE GUIDELINES FOR THE Psychiatric Evaluation of Adults

THIRD EDITION

Guidelines and Implementation

GUIDELINE I. Review of Psychiatric Symptoms, Trauma History, and Psychiatric Treatment History

Guideline Statements

Statement 1. APA recommends (1C) that the initial psychiatric evaluation of a patient include review of the patient's mood, level of anxiety, thought content and process, and perception and cognition.
Statement 2. APA recommends (1C) that the initial psychiatric evaluation of a patient include review of the patient's trauma history.
Statement 3. APA recommends (1C) that the initial psychiatric evaluation of a patient include review of the following aspects of the patient's psychiatric treatment history:

- Past and current psychiatric diagnoses
- Past psychiatric treatments (type, duration, and, where applicable, doses)
- Adherence to past and current pharmacological and nonpharmacological psychiatric treatments
- Response to past psychiatric treatments
- History of psychiatric hospitalization and emergency department visits for psychiatric issues[1]

Rationale

The goal of this guideline is to improve the quality of the doctor-patient relationship, the accuracy of psychiatric diagnoses, and the appropriateness of treatment selection.

The strength of research evidence supporting this recommendation is low. No prospective studies have addressed whether outcomes such as diagnostic accuracy and appropriate treatment planning are improved when the initial psychiatric evaluation includes review of psychiatric symptoms, trauma history, and psychiatric treatment history. Despite this, there is consensus by experts that the potential benefits described above clearly outweigh the potential harms.

The process of determining a patient's psychiatric diagnosis is complex (American Psychiatric Association 2013b). It requires knowledge of whether a patient is experiencing specific symptoms or exhibiting specific signs. Diagnostic accuracy also requires gathering information about the temporal development and duration of those signs and symptoms. For trauma-related diagnoses, as well as for neurocognitive disorders that are due to traumatic brain injury, the presence of a trau-

---

[1] As recommended in "Guideline III: Assessment of Suicide Risk" and "Guideline IV: Assessment of Risk for Aggressive Behaviors."

matic event is a precondition of diagnosis. Past trauma can also be a risk factor for the development of other diagnoses such as depressive or anxiety disorders (Hovens et al. 2012). A significant proportion of individuals with psychiatric illnesses appear to have experienced traumatic events (Coverdale and Turbott 2000; Cusack et al. 2004; Frueh et al. 2005; Lu et al. 2013; Oram et al. 2013; Posner et al. 2008), but trauma-related diagnoses such as posttraumatic stress disorder are often overlooked (Mueser et al. 1998). Thus, it is intuitively obvious that reviewing a patient's trauma history is essential to diagnostic accuracy. Knowledge of prior psychiatric diagnoses can also inform current diagnosis, since a patient may be presenting with a continuation of the prior disorder or may now have a different disorder that commonly co-occurs with the first (Gadermann et al. 2012; Kessler and Wang 2008; Kessler et al. 2005; Lenzenweger et al. 2007). The relevance of past treatments to diagnostic accuracy is more indirect but still relevant. If a patient has not responded to the primary treatments for a given diagnosis, it may suggest a need to reconsider the accuracy of that diagnosis. Treatment-emergent symptoms and signs (e.g., hypomania or mania in a depressed patient) may also require reassessment of the diagnosis.

Selecting an appropriate treatment will be an outgrowth of the patient's diagnosis as determined during the psychiatric evaluation; however, it also requires knowledge of the patient's current symptoms, trauma history, and previous diagnoses and psychiatric treatment experiences. The elements of the treatment plan will vary depending on the individual needs and preferences of the patient but will generally include treatment that addresses the patient's primary and co-occurring diagnoses. Often co-occurring psychiatric symptoms are present that are subthreshold or subsyndromal or may not respond to the treatment for the primary disorder (e.g., psychotic symptoms in mood disorders, cognitive impairment in schizophrenia). Such symptoms may contribute to functional impairments or risk of relapse and may also require specific intervention. Prior diagnoses of a co-occurring personality disorder may signal a need for a differing approach to psychotherapy than in an individual without such comorbidity. For individuals with a past trauma, this experience may influence their ability to establish a trusting relationship, and this may need to be considered in terms of the therapeutic alliance.

Recommended treatments also need to be feasible and tolerable as well as to show a preponderance of benefit over harm for the patient. Information about the patient's past treatment provides information on the prior benefits and tolerability of specific interventions but may also be relevant to the likely benefits and adverse effects of similar treatments. However, judgments about therapeutic benefits will need to be shaped by information on the adequacy of the treatment trial. For example, a different treatment or combination of treatments may be needed if a patient's symptoms do not respond to an adequate dose and duration of a medication or to an evidence-based psychotherapy delivered with high fidelity and for adequate duration. If a pattern of treatment resistance is identified, possible contributors need to be assessed and more aggressive treatment instituted to optimize the patient's functional outcomes.

Information on treatment-related side effects can be important in predicting the tolerability and safety of future treatment (e.g., agranulocytosis with clozapine, neuroleptic malignant syndrome or severe dystonic reactions with antipsychotic medication). Similarly, if adherence has been difficult for the patient in the past, it may suggest difficulties with the tolerability or feasibility of a particular treatment that would need to be addressed as part of the current treatment plan. Some treatments may be less likely to benefit the patient or more likely to be harmful to the patient depending on his or her prior psychiatric diagnoses or comorbidities (e.g., antidepressants in depressive episodes that occur in the context of bipolar disorder, use of bupropion in patients with an eating disorder).

Potential Benefits and Harms

In an initial psychiatric evaluation, there are a number of reasons that it is potentially beneficial to determine whether or not the patient has been experiencing abnormalities of mood, anxiety, thought content, thought process, and perception and cognition. Such signs and symptoms are important in first developing a differential diagnosis and then determining whether or not criteria for a specific DSM diagnosis have been met. Even when symptoms are subsyndromal, they may suggest the presence of additional co-occurring conditions or signal a need for additional treatment to address residual manifestations of illness. The pattern and presence of particular signs and symptoms is often important in considering the potential benefits and risks of treatment options. Baseline data may also be useful in interpreting signs and symptoms that develop during the course of treatment, either related to emergence or progression of underlying psychiatric disorders or as side effects of treatments. There are no plausible harms to determining if the patient is experiencing specific psychiatric signs or symptoms.

Determining whether or not the patient has a history of trauma is also important. Although most traumatized individuals will not develop psychopathology in the aftermath of a trauma, acute stress disorder or posttraumatic stress disorder may be part of the differential diagnosis when trauma-exposed individuals present for a psychiatric assessment. Regardless of whether or not a trauma-related disorder is present, past trauma may need to be specifically addressed as a part of the treatment. Given the emotional impact of traumatic events on individuals, many patients feel relieved to be able to discuss traumatic experiences when these are raised in a sensitive manner. However, it is also possible that raising questions about trauma could cause distress to some patients.

Obtaining information about current and previous psychiatric diagnoses can often be critical in formulating a differential diagnosis. Choosing among treatment options can be aided by determining whether a patient has already had a trial of a particular treatment. If a treatment has been tried in the past, knowledge of the patient's response, including therapeutic benefits and side effects, is relevant to determining whether an additional trial is warranted. In interpreting information about the patient's response, knowledge of the patient's adherence is also important as are specific aspects of treatment (e.g., type, duration, dose).

Assessment of psychiatric symptoms and psychiatric treatment history is by definition a core activity of an initial psychiatric evaluation. Other core activities include identifying the reason that the patient is presenting for evaluation and understanding the patient's background, relationships, life circumstances, and strengths and vulnerabilities. Each of these elements can be affected if a patient has been exposed to trauma. As a result, it is not possible to separate the cost of assessment of these domains from the overall cost of the evaluation itself, which will vary depending on the patient, the setting, and the model of payment.

Implementation

As described in the definition of "assessment" (see Glossary of Terms), there are a variety of ways that clinicians may perform these recommended assessments. Typically, a psychiatric evaluation involves a direct interview between the patient and the clinician. The specific approach to the interview will depend on many factors, including the patient's ability to communicate, degree of cooperation, illness severity, and ability to recall historical details. In some circumstances, questions on a particular topic (e.g., traumatic experiences) may cause the patient significant distress and may have to be pursued at a later session. Sensitivity may also be needed if a patient has experienced a traumatic event such as physical or sexual assault, because this can influence the ability to establish trust within the therapeutic relationship. Factors such as the patient's vocabulary and cultural background (American Psychiatric Association 2013a; Thombs et al. 2007) can also influence the patient's understanding and interpretation of questions and may require additional sensitivity on the part of the interviewer. Patients with intellectual disability or neurocognitive disorders may have difficulty in understanding questions as initially posed. In older individuals, difficulty understanding questions may signal unrecognized impairments in cognition or in hearing that require more detailed assessment. Flexibility may also be needed to frame questions in a clearer manner. At times (such as an evaluation of a patient with severe psychosis or dementia), obtaining information on psychiatric symptoms and history may not be possible through direct questioning.

When available, prior medical records, electronic prescription databases, and input from other treating clinicians can raise previously unknown information. Such sources can also be used to add details or corroborate information obtained in the interview. Family members, friends and other individuals involved in the patient's support network can be important sources of collateral information about the reason for evaluation, the patient's current symptoms and behavior, and past history, including trauma exposure and psychiatric treatment. Additional information such as knowledge of the patient's premorbid personality and level of function can help in identifying co-occurring disorders, including neurodevelopmental disorders, and in interpreting the onset and temporal course of the patient's illness. Communicating with family members or other caretaking persons can be particularly important when the patient requires assistance or supervision because of impaired function, unstable behavior, or neurocognitive impairment. Communication as part of the initial evaluation can also lay the groundwork for collaborating with the patient and involved family members in planning for and educating them about treatment. The extent of collateral interviews and review of prior records will be commensurate with the purpose of the evaluation, the complexity of the clinical presentation, and the diagnostic and therapeutic goals. For example, in an acute setting, collateral information may be crucial to developing an understanding of the patient's clinical condition, whereas in long-term outpatient psychotherapy it would be important to consider potential effects on the therapeutic relationship before obtaining collateral information from family or others. Except when immediate safety concerns are paramount, the confidentiality of the patient should be respected. In general, the default position is to maintain confidentiality unless the patient gives consent to a specific intervention or communication. At the same time, it is permissible for the clinician to listen to information provided by family members and other important people in the patient's life, as long as confidential information is not provided to the informant.

In some clinical contexts, such as a planned outpatient assessment, patients may be asked to complete an electronic- or paper-based form that inquires about psychiatric symptoms and key elements of the psychiatric history. Such forms may be completed prior to the visit or on arrival at the office and can serve as a starting point to explore reported symptoms or historical information. As an example of such a form, the DSM-5 Level 1 Cross-Cutting Symptom Measure (American Psychiatric Association 2013b) can be a useful tool to aid in the assessment of symptoms that may occur across different psychiatric diagnoses. The tool may be used both during an initial psychiatric evaluation and for subsequent monitoring. A self-report measure exists for adults and for children ages 11–17 years. A parent/guardian measure exists for children ages 6–17 years. Online versions of the measure are available at http://www.psychiatry.org/practice/dsm/dsm5/online-assessment-measures#Level1. Findings of the Level 1 measure can be amplified by follow-up questioning or the use of additional measures, such as the DSM-5 Level 2 Cross-Cutting Symptom Measures. To aid in the assessment of a patient's exposure to trauma, a brief self-report screening measure, the Trauma History Screen (Carlson et al. 2011), is available on request from the VA National Center for PTSD at http://www.ptsd.va.gov/professional/assessment/te-measures/ths.asp.

In addition to inquiring about the reason that the patient is seeking evaluation and learning about his or her current life circumstances, asking open-ended empathic questions about psychiatric symptoms is a common initial approach to the interview. This can be followed by more structured inquiry about specific symptoms (e.g., worries; preoccupations; changes in mood; suspicions; delusions or hallucinatory experiences; recent changes in sleep, appetite, libido, concentration, memory, or behavior): What is the severity of the patient's symptoms? Over what time course have these symptoms developed or fluctuated? Are associated features of specific psychiatric syndromes (i.e., pertinent positive or negative factors) present or absent during the present illness? What factors does the patient believe are precipitating, aggravating, or otherwise modifying the illness or are temporally related to its course? If suicidal or aggressive symptoms or behaviors are reported, these will also require further questioning to assess the patient's level of risk, as described in "Guideline III: Assessment of Suicide Risk" and "Guideline IV: Assessment of Risk for Aggressive Behaviors." Inquiry about specific symptoms may also be suggested by observations of the patient's behavior during the interview. For example, the presence of tremulousness might prompt questions about anxiety or about typical symptoms of alcohol or substance withdrawal.

Inquiring about a patient's trauma history also begins with open-ended and empathic questions. Individuals may differ in their perception of what constitutes a trauma. Asking about trauma in a non-specific fashion will help identify the experiences that had the greatest impact for the patient as well as provide an opportunity to learn about the patient's coping strengths and resilience in addressing past traumas. Information about traumas, including early adversity, may also be raised by the patient in the context of providing background information about his or his childhood upbringing, developmental history, school or occupational history, military history, relationship history, or family constellation. A history of childhood physical or sexual abuse is relatively common but may not be raised spontaneously by the patient unless specifically asked. Other follow-up questions about possible trauma will be suggested by other elements of the history (e.g., combat-related trauma in service members, migration stress in immigrants, posttraumatic symptoms relating to medical care in individuals who sustained a major injury or required intensive care).

In obtaining information about the past psychiatric history, questioning may vary in its level of detail at the initial meeting depending on the available time, the patient's recall of information, the patient's level of cooperation, and the complexity and urgency of clinical decision making. In many situations, the history of past diagnoses and treatments will need to be expanded at subsequent visits or augmented by history from other sources (e.g., prior clinicians, review of medical records). In terms of current and prior psychiatric diagnoses, information about principal and working diagnoses is relevant, when available, with specific attention to co-occurring psychiatric disorders, including neurodevelopmental disorders, neurocognitive disorders, substance use disorders, and personality disorders.

In reviewing prior trials of psychiatric treatment, the clinician may begin with open-ended questions about recent treatments, those that have been particularly helpful, and those that have been problematic. Follow-up questions could pursue more details on those treatments and then inquire about other treatments that have not yet been mentioned. Alternatively, a detailed longitudinal history of treatment can be obtained beginning with the patient's initial episode of illness and inquiring about each treatment in sequence. It is useful to inquire specifically about the full range of treatment settings (e.g., outpatient, partial hospital, inpatient) and treatment approaches, including psychotherapies, prescribed medications, electroconvulsive therapy (ECT), transcranial magnetic stimulation (TMS), self-help groups, 12-step programs, over-the-counter medications, herbal products, nutritional supplements, spiritual healers, and complementary or alternative treatment approaches. After the clinician has identified the category of treatment used, additional details are helpful to obtain depending on the type of treatment. Thus, for psychotherapies, it is useful to learn more about the format of therapy (e.g., individual, family, group), its type (e.g., supportive, cognitive-behavioral, interpersonal, psychodynamic, exposure with response prevention), the length and frequency of sessions, the duration of the course of therapy, and the quality of the relationship with the treating clinician. With pharmacological treatments (e.g., prescribed medications, over-the-counter medications, herbal products, nutritional supplements), information about the formulation, route, and dose and duration of treatment is important to obtain. With neurostimulatory treatments (e.g., ECT, TMS), the device type, treatment parameters, frequency of treatments, total number of treatments, and duration of the treatment course are important to know, including whether treatment included only an acute course or was followed by less frequent maintenance treatments. Similar information can be obtained for other forms of treatment. Regardless of the details of the treatment itself, it is important to determine how the patient responded to the treatment, in terms of both therapeutic benefits and side effects. When the clinician is inquiring about therapeutic benefits, it is useful to ask about symptom response and remission as well as changes in quality of life or levels of functioning and disability. For patients who did not respond to a specific treatment, the adequacy of treatment may depend on the clinical context (e.g., obsessive-compulsive disorder typically requires a higher dose of and a longer duration of treatment with a selective serotonin reuptake inhibitor than does major depressive disorder). Such details may be important in judging whether a patient's symptoms appear to be treatment resistant, with associated implications for treatment planning.

Typical side effects of treatment will vary with the treatment being used. Starting with open-ended questions about side effects with a particular treatment can help identify less common side effects that may have occurred and can also illuminate the kinds of side effects that may be of particular importance to the patient. With follow-up questions, the clinician can probe for more details and ask about more common adverse effects of a particular treatment, as indicated.

The clinician may also inquire in an open-ended fashion about the patient's adherence with previous treatments—for example, by asking about the patient's overall satisfaction with previous treatments and about any difficulties in taking medications (Velligan et al. 2010) or adhering to other forms of treatment. Problems with adherence in older individuals may signal early neurocognitive impairment that would warrant detailed cognitive assessment. Further questions can determine whether adherence problems are related to specific side effects of treatment, perceived lack of treatment benefits, personal beliefs about treatment (e.g., culturally related beliefs, personal preferences, family members' response to treatment, delusional ideas), or logistical barriers to treatment (e.g., cost, transportation to appointments, lack of child care). Depending on the clinical context, questions about adherence may extend to asking about court-ordered treatment programs.

These recommendations should not be viewed as representing a comprehensive set of questions relating to psychiatric assessment, nor should they be seen as an endorsement of a checklist approach to evaluation. Depending on the clinical setting, the patient's cooperation and ability to respond, the time available for the evaluation, and the type of treatment planned, some information may be more or less relevant to obtain as part of the initial assessment. The timing of the clinical event may also influence the need to obtain information at the initial interview as well as affect the level of detail that is required. With some information (e.g., severe medication side effects such as neuroleptic malignant syndrome), details are essential to obtain regardless of when the treatment may have occurred. Often, more recent symptoms, diagnoses, and details of treatment may be of greater relevance than those in the distant past.

The context and accuracy of the information obtained in the interview are also important to keep in mind before applying it to treatment planning. Simply asking about a patient's symptoms or history will not ensure that accurate or complete information is received. In some circumstances, the patient may minimize the severity or even the existence of his or her difficulties, particularly if help seeking is not voluntary. If observations of the patient's behavior during the interview or other aspects of the clinical presentation seem inconsistent with the patient's reported symptoms or history, additional questioning of the patient or others may be indicated. Factors such as time pressures, interviewing style, and clinician attitudes can also influence the ability to obtain accurate information during the assessment. Thus, the interviewer will want to be aware of his or her own emotions and reactions that may interfere with the evaluation process. Individuals also vary in their ability to recall details of diagnosis and treatment in an accurate manner. Gaps and inaccuracies in patient reports can arise from ordinary errors in comprehension, recall, and expression (Patten et al. 2012; Redelmeier et al. 2001; Simon et al. 2012). More errors occur when the patient is recalling more distant events (Patten et al. 2012; Simon et al. 2012). Factors other than time may also play a role in these variations in recall (Leikauf et al. 2013). For example, in older individuals, inconsistencies in the reported history may raise the possibility of a neurocognitive disorder that would warrant more detailed assessment of cognition.

Even when rigorous approaches are used to establish diagnoses, there may be shifts in the patient's diagnosis over time (Bromet et al. 2011; Mueller et al. 1999). Thus, the reported presence of a specific diagnosis in the past does not mean that the same diagnosis is accurate or persists. Issues with the accuracy of recall can also exist with respect to prior treatment (Simon et al. 2012). In addition, the patient's apparent therapeutic response, lack of response, or reported side effects may not be a direct result of the treatment itself. Rather, they may reflect the natural course of illness (e.g., transitioning to an episode of hypomania or mania), positive or negative life events, concomitant treatments (e.g., drug-drug interactions influencing serum levels, potential for augmenting effects of psychotherapies and medication), or other biologically mediated processes (e.g., cigarette use altering metabolism of prescribed medications).

Barriers to the use of these recommendations also exist, with a major barrier being constraints on clinician time and the need to assess many aspects of the patient's signs, symptoms, and history within a circumscribed period.

GUIDELINE II. Substance Use Assessment

Guideline Statements

APA recommends (1C) that the initial psychiatric evaluation of a patient include assessment of the patient's use of tobacco, alcohol, and other substances (e.g., marijuana, cocaine, heroin, hallucinogens) and any misuse of prescribed or over-the-counter medications or supplements.

Rationale

The goal of this guideline is to improve, during an initial psychiatric evaluation, the identification of patients with a substance use disorder and to facilitate treatment planning.

The strength of research evidence supporting this recommendation is low. A systematic search identified four studies that address the specific clinical question described under "Review of Supporting Research Evidence." The studies found that use of standardized questionnaires and collateral information can improve the identification of risky drinking, alcohol use disorders, and substance use compared with clinical interviews or routine care. All four studies were observational in design, and confounding factors were present in each. Furthermore, the applicability of the studies is limited. The studies mainly investigated the assessment of alcohol use, assessment did not necessarily occur in the context of a psychiatric evaluation, and the settings studied were not representative of the full range of settings in which psychiatric evaluations are performed.

Despite the low strength of this supporting research evidence, there is consensus by experts that assessing the patient's use of tobacco, alcohol, and other substances and misuse of prescribed or over-the-counter medications or supplements as part of an initial psychiatric evaluation has benefits that clearly outweigh the harms.

Additional indirect support for this recommendation comes from studies that have examined screening for tobacco and alcohol use in primary care and other medical settings. On the basis of a rigorous systematic review (Fiore et al. 2008), the U.S. Preventive Services Task Force (USPSTF) concluded that "the net benefits of tobacco cessation interventions in adults and pregnant women remain well established" (U.S. Preventive Services Task Force 2009, p. 551). Accordingly, the USPSTF recommends with high certainty of substantial benefit that clinicians should "ask all adults about tobacco use and provide tobacco cessation interventions for those who use tobacco products" and "ask all pregnant women about tobacco use and provide augmented, pregnancy-tailored counseling for those who smoke" (U.S. Preventive Services Task Force 2009, p. 551). The USPSTF has also concluded "with moderate certainty that there is a moderate net benefit to screening for alcohol misuse and brief behavioral counseling interventions in the primary care setting for adults aged 18 years or older" (Moyer 2013, p. 212; see also Jonas et al. 2012a, 2012b). In addition, the American College of Obstetricians and Gynecologists (ACOG) recommends screening of pregnant women for smoking (American College of Obstetricians and Gynecologists 2010) and for at-risk drinking and alcohol dependence, with behavioral counseling provided if screening is positive (American College of Obstetricians and Gynecologists 2011). They also recommend screening pregnant women for opioid use (American College of Obstetricians and Gynecologists 2012). By extension, screening and behavioral counseling is very likely to be beneficial in psychiatric settings, although further research confirmation is needed. Finally, the substantial rates at which substance use disorders and other psychiatric disorders co-occur (Compton et al. 2007; Grant et al. 2004; Hasin et al. 2007; Huang et al. 2006; Smith et al. 2006) also imply that screening for alcohol and substance use disorders would be relevant to differential diagnosis. Treatment planning is also influenced by identification of co occurring substance use disorders and other psychiatric illnesses as well as detection of medical conditions that commonly co-occur with substance use.

Potential Benefits and Harms

Assessment of tobacco, alcohol, and other substance use during the initial psychiatric evaluation may improve identification of patients with substance use disorders, including substance intoxication or withdrawal. Ensuring that initial psychiatric evaluations include assessment of substance use may improve the clinician's differential diagnosis because substance use disorders, other psychiatric disorders, and other medical conditions may share similar presenting symptoms, including anxiety, depression, mania, and psychosis.

If assessment identifies the presence of a substance use disorder, interventions can be offered, and there may be reductions in associated morbidity and mortality, such as from cardiovascular, respiratory, or hepatic diseases; blood-borne and sexually transmitted infectious diseases; injuries from motor vehicle accidents and other trauma; or deaths from suicide. Patients' psychological and social functioning may also be improved. Depending on the substance being used, provision of appropriate interventions may be associated with reductions in problems such as unemployment, divorce, homelessness, and criminal behaviors.

Potential harms of assessment have not been a focus of study but are likely to be minimal. Identifying a patient as having a substance use disorder when one is not present could result in unneeded treatment. If a patient becomes anxious or annoyed by being asked about substance use, this could interfere with the therapeutic relationship between the patient and the clinician. The cost of assessing substance use is difficult to separate from the overall cost of an initial psychiatric evaluation, which varies depending on the patient, the setting, and the model of payment. Another potential consequence is that time used to focus on assessment of substance use could reduce time available to address other issues of importance to the patient or of relevance to diagnosis and treatment planning.

Implementation

The clinical approach to inquiring about a patient's use of tobacco, alcohol, and other substances will vary with the context of the evaluation and with the patient's presenting symptoms. Typically, questions will focus on current use, but past use may also be relevant in patients with current use or when past use influences planning of treatment (e.g., decision making about the prescription of medication with potential for misuse or addition of treatment to maintain remission from substance use disorder). The specific substances that are asked about may be licit and illicit and include but are not limited to tobacco, alcohol, caffeine, marijuana, cocaine, methamphetamine, club drugs, inhalants, hallucinogens, or heroin.

Questions about misuse of prescribed or over-the-counter medications or supplements can often be introduced while the clinician is taking a history of the patient's prescribed medications. Prescribed medications that may be prone to misuse include but are not limited to androgens, benzodiazepines, barbiturates, other sedative-hypnotics, muscle relaxants, and opiate medications. Over-the-counter medications or supplements that may be misused include but are not limited to dextromethorphan, diphenhydramine, chlorpheniramine, caffeine, nicotine replacements, laxatives, and creatine. Newer substances of abuse are continuing to emerge and are frequently available over the counter, with names such as "bath salts" or "spice" that can disguise their true nature as substances of abuse.

A straightforward, nonconfrontational and open-ended approach to questions will usually elicit the most accurate responses, although individuals may underestimate their level of use or be reluctant to discuss their use of substances. Factors such as time pressures and clinician attitudes can also influence the ability to conduct an accurate assessment. When the clinician is speaking with patients about their current life circumstances and the reasons they are presenting for evaluation, it can be useful to consider whether unrecognized alcohol or substance use may be contributing to their symptoms or associated with stressors such as recent medical problems, relationship conflicts, traumatic exposures, or school/occupational, financial or legal difficulties. This can also serve as an opening to raise questions about the presence of tobacco, alcohol, or substance use. Observations made during the interview can provide additional clues to possible use (e.g., an odor of cigarettes or alcohol on the patient's breath; physical stigmata of injection drug use; slurred speech or other evidence of substance intoxication; tremulousness, abnormal vital signs, or other indications of alcohol or substance withdrawal).

Flexibility may be needed in tailoring questions to the individual patient. Slang terms for abused substances may be better understood by patients than medical terminology, but the specific words that are chosen may need to vary depending on factors such as patient age, culture, or locality. Family members and others who are involved in the patient's life may be able to give information that helps to identify and corroborate the type and extent of alcohol or substance use. In addition to information from spouses or intimate partners, parents of adult children who are living at home may have observed changes in behavior associated with substance use. Conversely, adult children may have noted signs of alcohol or other substance use in their parents. For individuals who reside in sober houses or community residence programs, affiliated staff members may be able to provide additional information on the patient's alcohol and substance use.

Asking questions during the initial psychiatric interview can also be supplemented by the use of self-report rating scales such as the DSM-5 Self-Rated Level 1 Cross-Cutting Symptom Measure, with administration of the DSM-5 Level 2—Substance Use Measure if the patient gives a positive response on the Level 1 alcohol or substance use items (American Psychiatric Association 2013b). These measures are available online at http://www.psychiatry.org/practice/dsm/dsm5/online-assessment-measures. Other measurement-based approaches to asking questions about alcohol or substance use include but are not limited to screening tests such as the Alcohol, Smoking and Substance Involvement Screening Test (ASSIST; World Health Organization 2010); the Fagerström Test for Nicotine Dependence (Heatherton et al. 1991); the Alcohol Use Disorders Identification Test (AUDIT; Saunders et al. 1993), or its shortened form, the AUDIT-C (Bush et al. 1998); and the Drug Abuse Screening Test (DAST; Skinner 1982). In some circumstances, information from laboratory testing may be available that provides clues to substance use. Examples include urine toxicology, blood alcohol levels, and measures of substance metabolites or biological effects of alcohol use (e.g., abnormal liver function, mean corpuscular volume of erythrocytes). If the patient exhibits signs of intoxication or withdrawal, scales such as the Clinical Institute Withdrawal Assessment for Alcohol—Revised (CIWA-Ar; Sullivan et al. 1989) or the Clinical Opiate Withdrawal Scale (COWS; Wesson et al. 2002) can be used to document signs and symptoms and guide treatment. When a patient has evidence of tobacco, alcohol, or other substance use in response to screening measures, interview questions, or laboratory testing, additional follow-up questions will generally be needed. Depending on the substance(s) being used, it may be important to delineate the route, quantity, frequency, pattern, typical setting, and circumstances of use as well as self-perceived benefits and psychiatric and other consequences of use.

Barriers to carrying out an assessment for tobacco, alcohol, and other substance use include the time required for a thorough assessment and lack of certainty that information obtained will be of value in establishing a diagnosis (e.g., because patients may not provide full details about their substance use). In addition, clinicians may be reluctant to ask questions about tobacco, alcohol, or substance use if they fear that it will upset patients, if they lack the time or confidence in their ability to follow through with appropriate interventions, or if resources for treatment are unavailable in the community.

GUIDELINE III. Assessment of Suicide Risk

Guideline Statements

Statement 1. APA recommends (1C) that the initial psychiatric evaluation of a patient include assessment of the following:

- Current suicidal ideas, suicide plans, and suicide intent, including active or passive thoughts of suicide or death
- Prior suicidal ideas, suicide plans, and suicide attempts, including attempts that were aborted or interrupted
- Prior intentional self-injury in which there was no suicide intent
- Anxiety symptoms, including panic attacks
- Hopelessness
- Impulsivity
- History of psychiatric hospitalization and emergency department visits for psychiatric issues
- Current or recent substance use disorder or change in use of alcohol or other substances
- Presence of psychosocial stressors (e.g., financial, housing, legal, school/occupational or interpersonal/relationship problems; lack of social support; painful, disfiguring, or terminal medical illness)
- Current aggressive or psychotic ideas, including thoughts of physical or sexual aggression or homicide[2]
- Mood, level of anxiety, thought content and process, and perception and cognition[3]
- Past and current psychiatric diagnoses[3]
- Trauma history[3]

Statement 2. APA recommends (1C) that the initial psychiatric evaluation of a patient *who reports current suicidal ideas* include assessment of the following:

- Patient's intended course of action if current symptoms worsen
- Access to suicide methods, including firearms
- Patient's possible motivations for suicide (e.g., attention or reaction from others; revenge, shame, humiliation, delusional guilt, command hallucinations)
- Reasons for living (e.g., sense of responsibility to children or others, religious beliefs)
- Quality and strength of the therapeutic alliance
- History of suicidal behaviors in biological relatives

Statement 3. APA recommends (1C) that the initial psychiatric evaluation of a patient *who reports prior suicide attempts* includes assessment of the details of each attempt (e.g., context, method, damage, potential lethality, intent).

Statement 4. APA recommends (1C) that the clinician who conducts the initial psychiatric evaluation document an estimation of the patient's suicide risk, including factors influencing risk.

Rationale

The goal of this guideline is to improve, during an initial psychiatric evaluation, the identification of patients who are at increased risk for suicide.

The strength of research evidence supporting these recommendations is low. However, a substantial body of epidemiological, cohort, case-control, and psychological autopsy studies has shown

---

[2] As recommended in the "Guideline IV: Assessment of Risk for Aggressive Behaviors."

[3] As recommended in the "Guideline I: Review of Psychiatric Symptoms, Trauma History, and Psychiatric Treatment History."

associations between the risk factors described in this guideline and long-term relative risk of suicide or suicide attempts in populations (Arsenault-Lapierre et al. 2004; Assessment and Management of Risk for Suicide Working Group 2013; Baxter and Appleby 1999; Bertolote et al. 2004; Borges et al. 2010; Brown et al. 2000; Carroll et al. 2014; Cavanagh et al. 2003; Conner et al. 2001; Geulayov et al. 2012; Haney et al. 2012; Harris and Barraclough 1997; Hawton et al. 2013; Ilgen et al. 2013; Large et al. 2011c; Li et al. 2011; Liu and Miller 2014; Miller et al. 2013; Nock et al. 2008). Nevertheless, there is no evidence that assessment of any of these factors can predict suicide in an individual (Assessment and Management of Risk for Suicide Working Group 2013; Brown et al. 2000; Coryell and Young 2005; Goldstein et al. 1991; Haney et al. 2012; King et al. 2001; Large et al. 2011a, 2011b; Pokorny 1993). Similarly, no study has shown the ability of a specific rating scale or assessment instrument to predict suicide in an individual (Assessment and Management of Risk for Suicide Working Group 2013; Haney et al. 2012; O'Connor et al. 2013). Furthermore, the utility of any assessment depends on availability of an effective treatment for the identified disorder or risk factor. Despite these limitations of the available research evidence, there is consensus by experts that the benefits of assessing the factors described in statements 1, 2, and 3 in an initial psychiatric evaluation clearly outweigh the potential harms, including unclear costs.

Suicide and suicide attempts occur at an increased rate in individuals with psychiatric disorders (Assessment and Management of Risk for Suicide Working Group 2013; Baxter and Appleby 1999; Borges et al. 2010; Haney et al. 2012; Harris and Barraclough 1997; Hawton and van Heeringen 2009; Li et al. 2011; Nock et al. 2008), and more than 90% of persons who die by suicide satisfy the diagnostic criteria for one or more mental disorders (Arsenault-Lapierre et al. 2004; Bertolote et al. 2004; Cavanagh et al. 2003; Conner et al. 2001). Suicide is rare, even within populations with a specific, high-risk mental disorder, such as major depressive disorder. Nevertheless, when suicide occurs, it is a devastating outcome for patients, their families, their communities, and clinicians. Substantial morbidity also occurs because of suicide attempts and other suicide-related behaviors. Assessment is an essential first step in helping clinicians estimate the patient's risk for suicide and other suicidal behaviors. When a patient is judged to be at risk, the clinician may use information obtained during the evaluation to determine an appropriate treatment setting and formulate an individualized treatment plan that addresses specific modifiable risk factors and may include heightened observation.

Potential Benefits and Harms

Inquiring about suicidal thoughts and related risk factors during the initial psychiatric evaluation may improve identification of patients who are at increased risk of suicide. If suicidal thoughts or other modifiable risk factors are found, specific interventions may be able to reduce the patient's subjective distress, symptom level, and overall risk of death or self-injury.

There is no evidence that risk of suicide is increased by asking a patient about prior experiences, symptoms such as hopelessness, or current suicidal ideas or suicide plans. A detailed systematic review on screening for suicide risk in primary care settings also has not identified any serious harms (O'Connor et al. 2013); however, assessment could misidentify individuals as being at significant acute risk when they are not. This could result in unneeded treatment, hospitalization, or other consequences for patients. Just as it is not possible to predict which individuals will die by suicide, there is no way to predict which individuals would be incorrectly identified as being at significant acute risk and no way to estimate the potential magnitude of this harm.

The cost of a suicide assessment is difficult to separate from the overall cost of an initial psychiatric evaluation, but both are low relative to the cost of suicide and suicide-related morbidity. Depending on the clinical characteristics of the patient and constraints such as time and setting, clinicians may prioritize suicide risk assessment over other parts of the evaluation and be unable to address other issues in as much detail.

Documenting an estimation of a patient's suicide risk may improve a clinician's decision making about the patient's diagnosis and treatment plan and may improve coordination of the patient's treatment with other clinicians. Potential consequences include reducing time available to inquire about and document other, potentially more important findings of an evaluation.

Implementation

As described in the definition of "assessment" (see Glossary of Terms), there are a variety of ways clinicians may obtain recommended information about a patient's suicide risk during an initial psychiatric evaluation. Typically, an evaluation involves a direct interview between the patient and the clinician. In some circumstances (such as an evaluation of a patient with severe psychosis or dementia), obtaining information on history, symptoms, and current mental status may not be possible through direct questioning. With all patients, other sources of information, such as prior medical records, and other treating clinicians can be important in corroborating information obtained in the interview or in raising previously unknown information. Family members, friends, and others in the patient's support network may be able to provide information about the patient's past history, family history, current mental state, activities, and psychosocial crises or stressors. They may also have observed behavior or been privy to communications from the patient that suggest suicidal ideation, suicide plans, or suicide intentions. Such information can be obtained without the psychiatrist's revealing private or confidential information about the patient. In clinical circumstances in which sharing information is important to maintain the safety of the patient or others, it is permissible to share such information without the patient's consent.

In implementing these recommendations, the clinician should note that some terms and concepts do not have precise definitions. Time-based terms such as "current," "recent," or "past" are often used in clinical contexts without a clear meaning. The concepts of active and passive suicidal ideas are commonly used by clinicians to contrast a specific "active" suicidal thought with "passive" ideas such as indifference to an accidental demise, a wish for death, or a desire to fall asleep and not wake up. The concepts of "aborted" and "interrupted" suicide attempts have also been defined in several ways— for example, that the attempt is stopped prior to fatal injury (Crosby et al. 2011) or stopped before any injury occurs (Barber et al. 1998). When the clinician is questioning a patient about suicidal behaviors, the primary goal is to identify any suicidal behaviors in which an attempt is begun, recognizing that it may not be conceptualized by the patient as a suicide attempt if it was stopped or interrupted.

Many suicide risk factors, such as hopelessness, are difficult to assess in a standardized way. In practice, the clinician must apply knowledge of the individual patient's circumstances to formulate useful questions about such risk factors. It would be impossible to list all of the possible elements that may contribute to a reason for living, a psychosocial stressor, a way to access suicide means, or a motivation or plan for suicide. Consequently, the clinician will need to frame specific questions related to these topics based on other information that has already been gathered in the interview.

Flexibility is also needed in the way that specific information is elicited. For example, to determine the patient's intended course of action if current symptoms or psychosocial stressors worsen, it is important to know which symptoms (e.g., depression, hallucinations, chronic pain, insomnia) or stressors are most upsetting and how these may interact with other factors motivating suicide. However, it is also important to frame the question in a way that gives the patient hope or suggests ways of coping if symptoms were to worsen (e.g., developing a safety plan, strengthening support networks, providing education about ways to contact the clinician) and to determine the patient's level of comfort in accessing such strategies. It may be useful to include family or friends in building support and strengthening approaches to coping. In some individuals, suicidal ideas may be motivated by feelings such as loneliness, self-hatred, or a sense of being a burden, not belonging, feeling trapped, or having no purpose (Jobes 2012; Van Orden et al. 2010). Such psychologically painful thoughts may be difficult to share, particularly at an initial interview. Cultural factors are also important to consider when framing questions, since issues such as shame, guilt, or humiliation can be culturally mediated and influence a patient's risk or willingness to discuss suicidal thoughts or suicide plans. If the patient has family members, friends, or other social acquaintances who have died by suicide or made suicide attempts, this can affect the patient's level of comfort in discussing his or her own thoughts and feelings.

Throughout the assessment, clinical judgment is needed in synthesizing information and observations. For example, determining whether the patient shows an "increased use of alcohol or other substances" will require comparing patterns of use at two or more points and then determining if a clinically significant change has occurred. Affirmative answers to some questions will often suggest other important lines of inquiry. For example, if a patient reports impulsivity, the clinician may be led to inquire about traumatic brain injury or thoughts about harming others; if a patient reports a suicide attempt, the clinician may be led to ask about precipitants, preparatory behaviors, method, physical damage, degree of lethality, and subsequent treatment. Information obtained may be relevant across multiple domains of a psychiatric evaluation—for example, the specific content of a patient's suicidal thoughts may be relevant to the clinician's estimation of the patient's risk of aggressive behaviors in addition to his or her risk of suicide.

Determining the quality and strength of the therapeutic alliance is also a multifaceted clinical judgment. At an initial evaluation, information may be limited to behavioral observations such as whether the patient appears to be cooperative with the assessment and forthcoming in answers to questions in contrast to being sullen, guarded, irritable, or agitated. Information about the patient's prior treatment relationships and current attitudes toward treatment may also provide insights into whether an alliance is beginning.

When the clinician is communicating with the patient, it is important to remember that simply asking about suicidal ideas or other elements of the assessment will not ensure that accurate or complete information is received. Patients with intellectual disability or neurocognitive disorders may have difficulty in understanding questions as initially posed. In older individuals, difficulty understanding questions may signal unrecognized impairments in cognition or in hearing. Flexibility may be needed to frame questions in a clearer manner. In other circumstances, the patient may minimize the severity or even the existence of his or her difficulties, particularly if help seeking is not voluntary. If other aspects of the clinical presentation seem inconsistent with an initial denial of suicidal thoughts, additional questioning of the patient or others may be indicated. Factors such as time pressures, interviewing style, and clinician attitudes can also influence the ability to conduct an accurate assessment. Thus, the psychiatrist will want to be aware of his or her own emotions and reactions that may interfere with the interview process. Use of open-ended questions is also more conducive to capturing the nuances and narrative of the patient's concerns, with follow-up questioning as needed to hone in on additional details. These recommendations should not be viewed as representing a comprehensive set of questions relating to suicide risk assessment, nor should they be seen as an endorsement of a checklist approach to evaluation. They also should not be viewed as suggesting the use of a standardized scale to identify individuals at high suicide risk. Many such scales have been designed and studied. Scales may be useful clinically—for example, to assist the clinician in developing a thorough line of questioning or to open communication with patients about particular feelings or experiences. However, no scale has been shown to provide a numerical score with clinically useful predictive value (Assessment and Management of Risk for Suicide Working Group 2013; Haney et al. 2012; O'Connor et al. 2013). Furthermore, no study has shown an ability to use population-based risk factors or combinations of those risk factors to accurately predict patients who die by suicide (Assessment and Management of Risk for Suicide Working Group 2013; Brown et al. 2000; Coryell and Young 2005; Goldstein et al. 1991; Haney et al. 2012; King et al. 2001; Large et al. 2011a; Pokorny 1993). Accordingly, estimation of an individual patient's risk for suicide is ultimately a matter of clinician judgment that requires synthesizing the available information and deciding how to weigh the contributions of multiple factors in estimating the patient's overall risk.

In synthesizing and documenting information gained from the initial evaluation, the clinician will focus primarily on estimating the patient's immediate suicide risk, while also considering longer-term contributors to risk that may need to be considered in treatment planning. Depending on the setting, if risk is judged to be elevated, the focus of the interview may shift to address the patient's safety, such as strengthening the patient's support network, developing a safety plan, or arranging for hospitalization.

In the context of suicidal behaviors, risk factors and protective factors interact in complex ways (Kraemer et al. 1997). When the clinician is estimating suicide risk and developing a plan to address it, it is helpful to distinguish between nonmodifiable risk factors and modifiable risk factors. The epidemiological concepts of distal and proximal risk factors can also help clinicians in thinking about suicide risk (Mościcki 2001). *Distal* risk factors reflect underlying vulnerabilities and predispositions, while *proximal* risk factors reflect more immediate precipitants or "triggers" for suicidal behaviors. Although proximal and distal risk factors may each be modifiable, they may require different types of interventions to address risk. Examples of nonmodifiable risk factors include demographic variables such as age and sex and factors related to clinical history such as past hospitalizations, past suicidal behaviors, childhood abuse, history of trauma, loss of a child, or family history of suicide or psychiatric illness. Although these factors are immutable, their relative impact on suicide risk may vary. For example, the relative risk of suicide can change as a person ages, with particularly high risk seen in white males over the age of 65. The risk associated with a prior hospitalization or prior suicide attempt is highest in the weeks to months after the event, but such events still confer some increased risk months or years later. Individuals with multiple suicide attempts or hospitalizations have additional increases in static risk. When there is a history of suicidal ideas, risk may vary depending on the worst-ever suicidal ideas. Learning about the ways in which the patient kept from acting on suicidal ideas can provide clues about available coping strategies as a protective factor. Where there is a history of suicide attempts, aborted or interrupted attempts, or other self-harming behavior, the patient's estimated risk can be modulated by other features of the suicidal behavior (e.g., psychosocial context, precipitating thoughts, presence of intoxication, timing, method, intent, consequences). Factors such as an early age at onset of depression or impulsive-aggressive traits, in combination with family history, can also be a marker of underlying vulnerability and risk (Mann et al. 2009). Psychiatric diagnoses and serious medical conditions, particularly those that are chronic, debilitating, disfiguring, or painful, can also contribute to an increase in the long-term relative risk of suicide (Assessment and Management of Risk for Suicide Working Group 2013; Baxter and Appleby 1999; Harris and Barraclough 1997; Haney et al. 2012; Hawton and van Heeringen 2009; Ilgen et al. 2013; Li et al. 2013; Nock et al. 2008). Again, the extent of risk can vary depending on factors such as illness severity, recency of diagnosis, and the number of comorbid conditions that are present. Among psychiatric disorders, mood disorders, psychotic disorders, anxiety disorders, posttraumatic stress disorder, substance use disorders, and disorders associated with impulsivity are most often associated with increased risk.

Most patients will also have one or more modifiable factors, superimposed on the nonmodifiable risk factors described above, that influence their suicide risk. Some of these factors are indications of an underlying or newly identified psychiatric disorder and can be reduced by treating the disorder itself or through targeted treatment of the specific sign or symptom. Examples of such signs and symptoms that can influence risk include psychosis, mood changes, hopelessness, insomnia, irritability, agitation, aggressive behaviors, and increases in substance use. In terms of suicidal ideas, the clinician will generally assign a higher level of risk to patients who have high degrees of suicide intent or describe more detailed and specific suicide plans, particularly those involving accessible means and violent irreversible methods. Psychosocial stressors may serve as precipitants to suicidal behaviors. Examples include lack of social support; stress relating to immigration; bereavement; problematic relationships (e.g., family members, intimate partners, friends, co-workers); and financial, housing, legal, or school/occupational problems. Other stressors may be relevant to certain groups of patients (e.g., military service members) (Assessment and Management of Risk for Suicide Working Group 2013). These stressors may be modifiable to some degree, but they also may be ongoing contributors to risk.

Individuals also have a unique balance between their personal motivations for suicide on the one hand and their reasons for living on the other hand. Motivations for suicide can include factors such as revenge, shame, humiliation, delusional guilt, command hallucinations, gaining attention or reaction from others, escaping physical or psychological pain, loneliness, self-hatred, or a sense of being a burden, not belonging, feeling trapped, or having no purpose. In contrast, reasons for living can include factors such as religious beliefs, sense of responsibility to children or others, plans for the future, or a sense of purpose in life. A strong social support network can also serve as a protective factor.

Given the large number of factors that can affect the risk of suicide, the clinician can neither review nor document all possible factors that could conceivably influence suicide risk. Rather, the clinician provides an estimated level of suicide risk, including factors that influence risk. It may also be helpful to conceptualize the overall risk in terms of underlying nonmodifiable risk factors as well as more immediate precipitants that may contribute to acute risk but are more likely to be modifiable. In addition to supporting clinical decision making and communication, such documentation can also serve as a foundation for planning of treatment. When recommendations are being implemented, a common barrier consists of constraints on clinician time and the need to assess many aspects of the patient's symptoms and history within the time available for the evaluation. Depending on the setting and clinical characteristics of the patient, the clinician may judge some parts of the evaluation as being of greater value in addressing safety concerns and planning initial treatment.

GUIDELINE IV. Assessment of Risk for Aggressive Behaviors

Guideline Statements

Statement 1. APA recommends (1C) that the initial psychiatric evaluation of a patient include assessment of the following:

- Current aggressive or psychotic ideas, including thoughts of physical or sexual aggression or homicide
- Prior aggressive or psychotic ideas, including thoughts of physical or sexual aggression or homicide
- Past aggressive behaviors (e.g., homicide, domestic or workplace violence, other physically or sexually aggressive threats or acts)
- Legal or disciplinary consequences of past aggressive behaviors
- History of psychiatric hospitalization and emergency department visits for psychiatric issues
- Current or recent substance use disorder or change in use of alcohol or other substances
- Presence of psychosocial stressors
- Exposure to violence or aggressive behavior, including combat exposure or childhood abuse
- Past or current neurological or neurocognitive disorders or symptoms

Statement 2. When it is determined during an initial psychiatric evaluation that the patient has aggressive ideas, APA recommends (1C) assessment of the following:

- Impulsivity, including anger management issues
- Access to firearms
- Specific individuals or groups toward whom homicidal or aggressive ideas or behaviors have been directed in the past or at present
- History of violent behaviors in biological relatives

Statement 3. APA suggests (2C) that the clinician who conducts the initial psychiatric evaluation should document an estimation of risk of aggressive behavior (including homicide), including factors influencing risk.

Rationale

The goal of this guideline is to improve, during an initial psychiatric evaluation, the identification of patients at risk for aggressive behaviors.

The strength of research evidence supporting this guideline is low. A substantial body of epidemiological, cohort, and case-control studies has shown associations between the risk factors described in this guideline and medium- to long-term relative risk of aggression in populations (Coid et al. 2006; Doyle and Dolan 2006; Doyle et al. 2012; Elbogen and Johnson 2009; Elbogen et al. 2006; Eriksson et al. 2011; Falk et al. 2014; Harford et al. 2013; Swanson et al. 1990; Ten Have et al. 2014; Van Dorn et al. 2012; Whittington et al. 2013; Witt et al. 2013). However, there is no evidence that assessment of any of these factors can predict aggression in an individual (Buchanan et al. 2012; Fazel et al. 2012; Large et al. 2011b; Rossegger et al. 2013; Singh et al. 2011, 2014; Thomas et al. 2005). Similarly, no study has supported the ability of a specific rating scale to predict aggression in an individual. Furthermore, the utility of any assessment depends on availability of an effective treatment for the identified disorder or risk factor. Despite these limitations of the available research evidence, there is consensus by experts that the benefits of assessing the factors described in statements 1 and 2 in an initial psychiatric evaluation clearly outweigh the potential harms, including unclear costs.

Potential Benefits and Harms

Inquiring about aggressive and homicidal thoughts and related risk factors during the initial psychiatric evaluation may improve identification of patients who are at increased risk of aggressive behaviors. If aggressive and homicidal thoughts or other modifiable risk factors are found, specific interventions may be able to reduce the patient's subjective distress and diminish the overall risk of harm. For example, assessment may help the clinician to determine an appropriate treatment setting and formulate an individualized treatment plan that may include heightened observation or may target specific modifiable risk factors.

There is no evidence that risk of aggression is increased by asking a patient about prior experiences, symptoms such as impulsivity, or current aggressive and homicidal ideas or plans; however, assessment could identify individuals as being at risk when they are not. This could result in unneeded treatment or hospitalization or other consequences for patients. Just as it is not possible to predict which individuals will exhibit aggressive behaviors, there is no way to predict which individuals would be incorrectly identified as being at risk and no way to estimate the potential magnitude of this harm.

The cost of assessing aggression is difficult to separate from the overall cost of an initial psychiatric evaluation, but both are low relative to the costs and harms of aggressive or homicidal behaviors. Depending on the clinical characteristics of the patient and constraints such as time and setting, clinicians may prioritize assessment of aggression risk over other parts of the evaluation and be unable to address other issues in as much detail.

Documenting an estimation of a patient's aggression risk may improve a clinician's decision making about the patient's diagnosis and treatment plan and may improve coordination of the patient's treatment with other clinicians. As noted above, potential harms could include reducing time available to document other, potentially more important findings of an evaluation.

Implementation

As described in the definition of "assessment" (see Glossary of Terms), there are a variety of ways clinicians may obtain recommended information about a patient's aggression risk during an initial psychiatric evaluation. Typically, an evaluation involves a direct interview between the patient and the clinician. In some circumstances (e.g., during an evaluation of a patient with severe psychosis or dementia), obtaining information on history, symptoms, and current mental status may not be possible through direct questioning. With all patients, other sources of information can be important in corroborating information obtained in the interview or in raising previously unknown information. When available, prior medical records, input from other treating clinicians, and information from family members or friends can provide added details on issues such as recent symptoms, stressors, past history, and family history. Because aggression may have genetic patterns, "family history" should be understood to include any history of abuse or violence in the patient's biological relatives. Exposure to violence by nonbiological family members can also be important to consider.

When the clinician is communicating with the patient, it is important to remember that simply asking about aggressive ideas or other elements of the assessment will not ensure that accurate or complete information is received. Patients with intellectual disability or neurocognitive disorders may have difficulty in understanding questions as initially posed. In older individuals, difficulty understanding questions may signal unrecognized impairments in cognition or in hearing. Such individuals may also become more agitated when feeling overwhelmed or overloaded with cognitive demands. Flexibility may be needed to frame questions in a clearer and simpler manner. In other circumstances, the patient may minimize the severity or even the existence of his or her difficulties, particularly if help seeking is not voluntary. If other aspects of the clinical presentation seem inconsistent with an initial denial of aggressive thoughts or prior aggressive behaviors, additional questioning of the patient or others may be indicated. Factors such as time pressures, interviewing style, and clinician attitudes, including concern for personal safety, can also influence the ability to conduct an accurate assessment. Thus, the psychiatrist will want to be aware of his or her own emotions and reactions that may interfere with the interview process and also attend to his or her own safety as well as that of the patient.

Some terms and concepts used in this guideline are impossible to define precisely. Time-based terms such as "current," "recent," or "prior" are often used in clinical contexts without a clear meaning. Many aggression risk factors, such as impulsivity, would be difficult or even impossible to assess in a standardized way. A progressive sequence of open-ended questions is more conducive to capturing the nuances and narrative of the patient's concerns and can often provide a starting point for further discussion (e.g., What types of situations can trigger you to become angry? When you do become angry, do you lose your temper easily? How often do angry urges happen and how long do they last? Do you ever get so angry that you feel like you want to hurt someone? Do you ever daydream about hurting others? Are there specific individuals who you have thought of hurting? What helps you calm down when you are feeling angry? What ways do you use to keep yourself from acting on your angry impulses?). Understanding the reasons that the patient is presenting for evaluation is also important in determining the interpersonal and psychosocial context in which aggressive thoughts might arise.

In practice, clinicians must also apply knowledge of the individual patient's circumstances to formulate useful questions about risk factors for aggression. For example, firearms may be readily available in some geographic regions or with some occupations. Relevant psychosocial stressors may commonly include housing problems or homelessness, financial stresses, job loss, relationship loss, or lack of social support but may also include other stressors that are particularly salient for a given individual (e.g., public humiliation, victim of violence or bullying, custody disputes or spousal estrangement, grievance against a specific person, including past or current clinicians). In addition, the clinician will need to frame specific questions based on other information that has already been gathered in the interview. Inquiring about legal or disciplinary consequences of aggressive behaviors, such as school expulsions, warrants, arrests, jail or prison sentences, probation, parole or orders of protection, would depend on the answers to prior questions. When aggressive behaviors have occurred, it is often helpful to learn about the context of those events (e.g., setting; precipitants; object of violence, including other people or animals; cultural mediators of behavior, including gang membership; associated use of substances or potentially disinhibiting medications; subsequent callousness or remorse). In terms of neurological disorders, common concerns would include traumatic brain injury (Fazel et al. 2009b), but other information from the history or interview may suggest other possible conditions, such as intellectual disability or neurocognitive disorders.

Clinical judgment may also be needed in synthesizing information and observations from the interview. For example, determining whether the patient shows an "increased use of alcohol or other substances" will require a comparison of patterns of use at two or more points and then determining if a clinically significant change has occurred. Diagnostic considerations can also be relevant, because research studies have identified diagnostic subgroups, such as individuals with substance use disorders or antisocial personality disorder, who show an increased relative risk of aggression on a long-term basis in community settings (for more information, see Coid et al. 2006; Doyle and Dolan 2006; Doyle et al. 2012; Elbogen and Johnson 2009; Elbogen et al. 2006; Eriksson et al. 2011; Falk et al. 2014; Harford et al. 2013; Swanson et al. 1990; Ten Have et al. 2014; Van Dorn et al. 2012). Individuals in other settings, including psychiatric inpatient or forensic units, or with specific diagnoses may show somewhat different patterns of risk factors (Cornaggia et al. 2011; Dack et al. 2013; Douglas et al. 2009; Doyle et al. 2012; Fazel et al. 2009a, 2010), with substantial variability across studies. In nursing home patients, a substantial proportion of individuals with neurocognitive disorders exhibit agitated or aggressive behaviors (Selbæk et al. 2013). Such behaviors are also a common precipitant for hospital admission when a neurocognitive disorder is present (Toot et al. 2013), requiring additional questions about concurrent medical conditions such as infections or recent medication changes.

For an individual patient, other factors may be relevant to clinical decision making about aggression risk. For example, for a patient whose psychiatric disorder is currently symptomatic, the severity of symptoms may be relevant as well as whether the patient is unusually angry or irritable during the evaluation, feels persecuted by an identified individual, or is experiencing command hallucinations to harm others. Whenever an individual has aggressive or homicidal ideas or behaviors, it is important to identify any intended targets of aggression. If a specific target is identified, the clinician will need to use his or her clinical judgment in deciding whether the patient requires a more supervised setting of care (to provide protection for the identified target and more intensive treatment for the patient) or whether the identified target should be warned of the potential for harm, or both. There is also considerable variability by state on the case law and statutes that address the Tarasoff duty to protect (Soulier et al. 2010), and the clinician will want to become familiar with the requirements of his or her local jurisdiction. Assessment of aggressive ideas will commonly be integrated with assessment for suicidal ideation, and if suicidal thoughts are identified, it is important to look for factors that might suggest a possible risk of murder-suicide.

Additional details on conducting a risk assessment for aggressive behaviors can be found in the APA's "Resource Document on Psychiatric Violence Risk Assessment" (Buchanan et al. 2012) and the supplemental materials posted on the *American Journal of Psychiatry* Web site (http://ajp.psychiatryonline.org/data/Journals/AJP/20334/340_ds001.pdf).

These recommendations should not be viewed as representing a comprehensive set of questions relating to aggression risk assessment, nor should they be seen as an endorsement of a checklist approach to evaluation. Although structured assessments of aggression risk have been developed and studied, none has sufficient predictive validity to identify individuals at high aggression risk in clinical settings (Buchanan et al. 2012; Fazel et al. 2012; Large et al. 2011b; Rossegger et al. 2013; Singh et al. 2011, 2014; Thomas et al. 2005). Accordingly, estimation of an individual patient's risk for aggression is ultimately a matter of clinician judgment that requires synthesizing the available information and deciding how to weigh the contributions of multiple factors, including those that may prevent the patient from acting on aggressive ideas. This clinical decision-making process and a discussion of the factors that are judged to influence the risk of aggressive behavior for the individual patient can be included as part of the clinical documentation, typically in a brief paragraph. Distinctions between modifiable risk factors (e.g., alcohol or substance use, psychosis) that could be reduced by treatment (Elbogen et al. 2006; Swanson et al. 2008) or other interventions and static, nonmodifiable risk factors (e.g., age, sex, clinical history) are also important to note in assessing and documenting risk and arriving at a plan for addressing it.

When recommendations are being implemented, a common barrier consists of constraints on clinician time and the need to assess many aspects of the patient's symptoms and history within the time available for the evaluation. Depending on the setting and clinical characteristics of the patient, the clinician may prioritize some parts of the evaluation and documentation process that are judged to have greater value in addressing safety concerns and planning initial treatment.

GUIDELINE V. Assessment of Cultural Factors

Guideline Statements

Statement 1. APA recommends (1C) that the initial psychiatric evaluation of a patient include assessment of the patient's need for an interpreter.

Statement 2. APA recommends (1C) that the initial psychiatric evaluation of a patient include assessment of cultural factors related to the patient's social environment.

Statement 3. APA suggests (2C) that the initial psychiatric evaluation of a patient include assessment of the patient's personal/cultural beliefs and cultural explanations of psychiatric illness.

Rationale

The goal of this guideline is to improve, during an initial psychiatric evaluation, identification of cultural factors that could influence the therapeutic alliance, promote diagnostic accuracy, and enable appropriate treatment planning.

The strength of research evidence supporting this guideline is low. Despite this, there is consensus by experts that the benefits of including the assessments described in statements 1 and 2 in an initial psychiatric evaluation clearly outweigh the potential harms.

Individuals present for psychiatric assessment with a wide range of backgrounds, cultures, and beliefs. Data from the American Community Survey (U.S. Census Bureau 2012) show that the U.S. population is extremely diverse in its ancestry and racial and ethnic characteristics. About 13% of persons living in the United States were born in a different country, with about one-half of these individuals born in Latin America and about a one-quarter in Asia. Approximately one-fifth of the U.S. population, about 60 million individuals, speak a language other than English in their home. Of these individuals, slightly more than one-half also speak English very well. Nevertheless, increasing numbers of individuals in the United States have limited proficiency in English, which can affect their receipt of appropriate health care.

No study has specifically examined whether health outcomes are improved when an initial psychiatric evaluation includes assessment of the patient's language needs and culture. Available studies do suggest, however, that discordance between the patient's and the clinician's language or limitations in English proficiency challenge health-related communication, reduce diagnostic reliability, decrease the effectiveness of care, and heighten the risks of treatment in psychiatric (Bauer and Alegría 2010; Bauer et al. 2010; Kim et al. 2011; Leng et al. 2010) and nonpsychiatric (Fernandez et al. 2011; Wilson et al. 2005) settings. Furthermore, in nonpsychiatric settings, the use of professionally trained interpreters during the evaluation of patients with limited English proficiency has been found to reduce communication errors and enhance comprehension of medical information, health care utilization, clinical outcomes, and satisfaction with care (Karliner et al. 2007).

On the basis of this indirect research evidence and common sense, assessing a patient's need for an interpreter during an initial psychiatric evaluation is a necessary first step in promoting effective communication between the patient and the clinician. This is true even when the patient speaks the same language as the clinician. Some patients will speak more than one language and have differing levels of fluency in each. Verbal and written language fluency may be discordant, and comprehension may differ from spoken language fluency. Even when an interpreter is not used, knowledge of the patient's language ability may help the clinician tailor his or her communications appropriately—

for example, use vocabulary the patient understands or provide written educational materials in the patient's preferred language and at his or her reading level.

Factors such as age, ethnicity, gender, race, religion, and sexuality can shape a patient's personal and cultural identity as well as influence his or her communications with mental health professionals. Some of these factors, including sex, race, ethnicity, and sexual orientation, have been found to be associated with disparities in medical care and health outcomes (Gone and Trimble 2012; Hall-Lipsy and Chisholm-Burns 2010; Lagomasino et al. 2005; Primm 2006; Smedley et al. 2003; Thomas et al. 2011; Vega et al. 2009).

Individuals from different backgrounds may also differ in their explanations of illness, views of mental illness, and preferences for psychiatric treatment, particularly given the cross-cultural differences in the stigma of psychiatric disorders (Abdullah and Brown 2011; Angermeyer and Dietrich 2006; Jimenez et al. 2012; Lim et al. 2015). For example, an individual's self concept, response to stressors, or current symptomatology may be shaped by racism, sexism, or discrimination; by traumatic experiences during or after migration from other countries; or by challenges of acculturation, such as intergenerational family conflict. Cultural factors can also influence the patient's style of relating with authority figures such as health care professionals. The relevance of cultural factors to both diagnosis and treatment suggests potential benefits of identifying personal and cultural factors and integrating that understanding into the provision of care, including psychoeducation and other interventions to address culturally related stigma and shame. Such an approach has been recommended by experts (Mezzich et al. 2009; Yamada and Brekke 2008) and organizations, including the APA (DSM-5 Cultural Formulation Interview; American Psychiatric Association 2013a), The Joint Commission (2010, 2011), and the Office of Minority Health of the U.S. Department of Health and Human Services (2014).

Clinicians can improve their ability to assess cultural factors that are relevant to diagnosis and treatment by using an assessment instrument such as the DSM-5 Cultural Formulation Interview and by learning about cultures that are represented among their patients (Lim et al. 2015).

Potential Benefits and Harms

In an initial psychiatric evaluation, the clinician typically gathers information about a patient through a face-to-face interview. There are obvious potential benefits to ensuring that the patient's need for an interpreter is assessed early in the evaluation. Use of an interpreter could improve the accuracy of diagnosis by allowing the patient to communicate nuances of his or her mental state and symptoms. It could also ensure the formulation and implementation of an appropriate treatment plan and assist the clinician in providing education about symptoms, potential treatments, and their possible side effects. There are no plausible harms of assessing the need for an interpreter, and the cost of the assessment seems negligible.

Similarly, the potential benefits of inquiring about a patient's cultural beliefs, cultural explanations of illness, and cultural factors related to his or her social environment during an initial psychiatric evaluation include promoting a therapeutic alliance, improving the accuracy of a diagnosis, and ensuring the formulation of an appropriate treatment plan. For example, for cultural reasons, a patient may consider some treatments to be particularly valuable and others unacceptable. Furthermore, interventions may be available that are designed for patients with a specific cultural background or that are designed to address disparities in the care of specific populations such as ethnic minorities (Grote et al. 2009). Knowledge of the patient's sociocultural environment may help the clinician to choose interventions that take advantage of the patient's existing networks of support.

Potential harms of a cultural assessment (e.g., if the assessment is done poorly) could include offending the patient and damaging the alliance. The cost of doing a cultural assessment is difficult to separate from the overall cost of an initial psychiatric evaluation, which varies depending on the patient, the setting, and the model of payment. When time is used to focus on cultural issues, the time available to address other issues of importance to the patient may be reduced.

Implementation

For many patients, language needs can be easily determined. For others, assessment may need to establish both the need for an interpreter and the appropriateness of different interpreter options. This may be apparent at the time an appointment is being scheduled, but it may also be identified as a need at the time of the initial visit. Although language-concordant physicians or trained in-person interpreters have typically been used (Locatis et al. 2010), telephonic and video-based options for accessing professional interpreters are increasingly available and offer greater patient privacy (Gany et al. 2007). However, remote interpreting services can be more challenging to use if patients speak softly or are unable to cooperate fully with the interview. Some individuals who are deaf or hard-of-hearing may prefer to communicate through an in-person or video-based sign language interpreter, whereas others prefer to communicate through other approaches (e.g., lip reading, face-to-face keyboards, writing) (Fellinger et al. 2012).

Psychiatrists and other mental health professionals may speak more than one language and may be able to communicate in the patient's preferred language. Even if the clinician is reasonably fluent in the patient's preferred language, there may be situations in which a trained interpreter may have a greater understanding of the nuances of the patient's communication. In addition to considering concordance of language per se, clinicians and interpreters will want to consider the effects that different dialects and uses of idiom can have in the communication process.

With respect to the assessment of a patient's culture, beginning with open-ended questions is likely to be more conducive to learning about the individual and his or her beliefs. These questions may flow naturally from the reasons that the patient presents for evaluation or may require more specific attention during the interview. An individualized approach is important because there is substantial heterogeneity of individual beliefs, including those related to cultural factors (Lim et al. 2015). Even the definition of cultural factors and personal/cultural beliefs is vague and broad in scope, with significant overlap with other biopsychosocial influences. Individuals within a specific cultural group will have a wide range of beliefs relating to that culture. Some patients will use culturally specific treatments, including medications, supplements, health practices, and consultation with culturally specific healers. Other treatments may be prohibited or misunderstood because of cultural beliefs. There is also substantial heterogeneity in the degree to which an individual patient may gain support or feel estranged from cultural networks, making it important to explore the patient's views and feelings. When present, cultural networks (e.g., religious affiliations, tribal supports, military command structure) can help to enhance a patient's social ties and supports. In many cultures, families play an important source of support during times of illness, and in some cultures treatment decisions are made by family members rather than by the individual. Family members or members of a patient's cultural group may also be helpful in explaining the patient's belief system and whether the patient's current beliefs and behaviors are at odds with it. Examples may include spiritual beliefs that are not part of an organized religion or cultural or religious rituals, including food preferences.

A number of barriers exist to conducting such an assessment, including underlying cultural biases of clinicians and the time needed to conduct a thorough exploration of culturally related beliefs, influences, and networks. Some clinicians are unsure of the value of assessing cultural factors or feel unskilled in conducting a complex assessment of this type. In some settings, elements of the assessment may be elicited by other mental health professionals and can serve as the starting point for the psychiatrist's evaluation. In other situations, the psychiatrist will wish to begin assessment of cultural factors at the initial evaluation, particularly as they relate to the patient's presenting problem. More detailed inquiry can then occur as the therapeutic relationship develops, the patient's sociocultural context changes, or other findings suggest the need for in-depth knowledge of the patient's culturally related beliefs.

For clinicians who lack experience in assessing cultural factors, the DSM-5 Cultural Formulation Interview (American Psychiatric Association 2013a) offers a semi-structured framework for initiating questioning relating to key elements of the cultural identity of the individual, cultural conceptualizations of distress, psychosocial stressors and cultural features of vulnerability and resilience, and cultural features of the relationship between the individual and the clinician. Depending on the patient's answers to initial questions in the interview, supplementary modules are available to guide detailed questioning.

GUIDELINE VI. Assessment of Medical Health

Guideline Statements

Statement 1. APA recommends (1C) that the initial psychiatric evaluation of a patient include assessment of whether or not the patient has an ongoing relationship with a primary care health professional.

Statement 2. APA recommends (1C) that the initial psychiatric evaluation of a patient include assessment of the following:

- General appearance and nutritional status
- Involuntary movements or abnormalities of motor tone
- Coordination and gait
- Speech, including fluency and articulation
- Sight and hearing
- Physical trauma, including head injuries
- Past or current medical illnesses and related hospitalizations
- Relevant past or current treatments, including surgeries, other procedures, or complementary and alternative medical treatments
- Allergies or drug sensitivities
- Sexual and reproductive history
- Past or current sleep abnormalities, including sleep apnea

Statement 3. APA recommends (1C) that the initial psychiatric evaluation of a patient include assessment of all medications the patient is currently or recently taking (i.e., both prescribed and nonprescribed medications, herbal and nutritional supplements, and vitamins) and the side effects of these medications.

Statement 4. APA suggests (2C) that the initial psychiatric evaluation of a patient also include assessment of the following:

- Height, weight, and body mass index (BMI)
- Vital signs
- Skin, including any stigmata of trauma, self-injury, or drug use
- Cardiopulmonary status
- Past or current endocrinological disease
- Past or current infectious disease, including sexually transmitted diseases, HIV, tuberculosis, hepatitis C, and locally endemic infectious diseases such as Lyme disease
- Past or current neurological or neurocognitive disorders or symptoms
- Past or current symptoms or conditions associated with significant pain and discomfort

Statement 5. In addition to a psychiatric review of systems,[4] APA suggests (2C) that the initial psychiatric evaluation of a patient include a review of the following systems:

- Constitutional symptoms (e.g., fever, weight loss)
- Eyes

---

[4] As recommended in "Guideline I: Review of Psychiatric Symptoms, Trauma History, and Psychiatric Treatment History."

- Ears, nose, mouth, throat
- Cardiovascular
- Respiratory
- Gastrointestinal
- Genitourinary
- Musculoskeletal
- Integumentary (skin and/or breast)
- Neurological
- Endocrine
- Hematological/lymphatic
- Allergic/immunological

Rationale

The goal of this guideline is to improve, during an initial psychiatric evaluation, identification of nonpsychiatric medical conditions that could affect the accuracy of a psychiatric diagnosis and the safety of a psychiatric treatment plan.

The strength of research evidence supporting statements 1, 2, and 3 is low. As described under "Review of Supporting Research Evidence," studies were identified that do address whether diagnostic accuracy is improved by physical assessment or a medical history, but these elements of the evaluative process were not examined as discrete interventions. The studies also did not address whether treatment safety is affected by physical assessment, medical history, review of medications, or review of systems, or whether diagnostic accuracy is affected by review of medications or review of systems. The lack of generalizability of these studies is an additional factor that weakens their strength. Despite this, there is consensus by experts that including the assessments described in statements 1, 2, and 3 in an initial psychiatric evaluation has benefits for diagnostic accuracy and treatment safety that clearly outweigh the potential harms.

Individuals with psychiatric disorders can have medical conditions that influence their functioning, quality of life, and life span. Relative to the general population, mortality rates are increased for individuals with mental illness, particularly those with psychotic disorders, depressive disorders, alcohol/substance use disorders, personality disorders, and delirium (Chang et al. 2010; Chwastiak et al. 2010; Fok et al. 2012; Haklai et al. 2011; Honkonen et al. 2008; Høye et al. 2013; Lemogne et al. 2013; Markkula et al. 2012; Witlox et al. 2010). Estimates suggest that the life span of an individual with a mental illness is approximately 8 years shorter than the life span of individuals in the general population (Druss et al. 2011). For individuals with serious mental illness, the reduction is even more dramatic: up to 25 years (Parks et al. 2006; Saha et al. 2007). Individuals with mental illness have increased cardiovascular mortality (Miller et al. 2006; Morden et al. 2012; Newcomer and Hennekens 2007; Osborn et al. 2007; Parks et al. 2006; Piatt et al. 2010; Roshanaei-Moghaddam and Katon 2009), greater incidence of medical conditions (Dickerson et al. 2006a; Kisely et al. 2008; Leucht et al. 2007; McGinty et al. 2012; Osborn et al. 2007), greater risk of injury (McGinty et al. 2013; Piatt et al. 2010), and greater rates of health risk factors such as obesity and tobacco use (Dickerson et al. 2006b; Lawrence et al. 2009; Osborn et al. 2006). Dental health is also poorer in those with severe mental illness (Kisely et al. 2011; Leucht et al. 2007) and can contribute to health risks such as community acquired pneumonia and endocarditis. Physical functioning is often reduced as well (Chafetz et al. 2006) and may be independently associated with mortality risk (Hayes et al. 2012). When individuals with a serious mental illness are diagnosed with medical conditions, they may be less aware of their concomitant disorders than individuals without a mental illness (Kilbourne et al. 2006). In addition, the quality and type of treatment they receive is frequently disparate from care received by the general population (Druss et al. 2011; Goldberg et al. 2007; Kilbourne et al. 2008; Kisely et al. 2011; Mitchell et al. 2009, 2012; Salsberry et al. 2005). Furthermore, some individuals with mental illness may be unable to understand and adhere to treatment for their illness.

These disparities in care for those with psychiatric illness worsen the morbidity and mortality due to medical conditions as compared with individuals in the general population.

Psychiatric and medical issues are interrelated in a number of other ways. Medical conditions can contribute to the genesis of psychiatric symptoms and syndromes (American Psychiatric Association 2013b; David et al. 2009) or can complicate the diagnosis of psychiatric disorders. For example, an individual with hyperthyroidism may develop symptoms of anxiety. A frontal lobe tumor may result in a mood syndrome or neurocognitive impairment. An individual with uremia or obstructive sleep apnea may feel apathetic, fatigued, and inattentive, wrongly implying the presence of depression even in the absence of mood changes.

Knowledge of the medications that a patient is taking is also important. Medications used to treat medical conditions can interact with psychotropic medications (Ferrando et al. 2010; Sinclair et al. 2010; Zorina et al. 2013). Many individuals receiving psychiatric treatment are taking multiple medications, and this magnifies the likelihood of drug-drug interactions (Haueis et al. 2011; Mojtabai and Olfson 2010; Sandson et al. 2005; Thomas et al. 2010). Patients may also be taking nonprescribed medications such as nutritional supplements or herbal products (Freeman et al. 2010; Meeks et al. 2007; Ravindran and da Silva 2013), which can interact with psychotropic medications, influencing therapeutic benefits or side effects. Side effects of somatic treatments for psychiatric conditions can also produce or increase the risks of preexisting medical conditions (Goldberg and Ernst 2012). Other medication effects can mask physical findings that are important to clinical decision making. For example, a beta-adrenergic receptor antagonist can blunt changes in vital signs (e.g., tachycardia, elevations in blood pressure) that signal alcohol or benzodiazepine withdrawal. In addition, medications can be associated with false positive results on toxicology testing (Brahm et al. 2010; Rengarajan and Mullins 2013) or modify other laboratory findings leading to an incorrect diagnosis. Lack of information or confusion about prescribed medications and dosages can also contribute to medical errors (Fitzgerald 2009; Procyshyn et al. 2010; Tully et al. 2009).

Given the above, an understanding of the patient's medical status is important to 1) properly assess the patient's psychiatric symptoms and their potential cause, 2) determine the patient's need for medical care, and 3) consider potential effects on the patient's medical conditions or related treatments when choosing among psychiatric treatments.

Potential Benefits and Harms

In an initial psychiatric evaluation, determining whether or not the patient has an ongoing relationship with a primary care health professional is potentially beneficial from several vantage points. In patients who are already receiving medical care, communication with the primary care professional could be useful in coordinating assessments and treatment. If the patient has had a recent medical assessment, the psychiatrist may be able to review the results of the history, physical examination, and laboratory or imaging findings in lieu of a direct assessment of the patient. Such information is often important in formulating a differential diagnosis and considering the benefits and risks of potential treatment options. There are no plausible harms to determining if the patient has a relationship with a primary care professional.

Similarly, there are many potential benefits to ensuring that the initial psychiatric evaluation includes assessment of the aspects of the patient's medical health listed in statement 2. Signs and symptoms of illness may be consistent with either a psychiatric disorder or another medical condition. Differential diagnosis can be aided by knowledge of past or current nonpsychiatric medical disorders. Previously unrecognized medical illnesses may also be identified and addressed directly or by referral to another clinician. Baseline data about medical conditions may be useful later in interpreting physical signs and symptoms that emerge in the course of treatment, either related to progression of underlying medical conditions or as side effects of psychiatric treatments.

The potential benefits of knowing the medications that a patient is taking are also multifaceted. Use of prescribed medications, over-the-counter medications, vitamins, nutritional supplements, and herbal products can be associated with psychiatric signs and symptoms that would be relevant to differential diagnosis. These medications can also interact with medications for psychiatric conditions and thereby influence treatment planning.

The cost of assessing these aspects of the patient's medical health is difficult to separate from the overall cost of an initial psychiatric evaluation, which varies depending on the patient, the setting, and the model of payment. When time within the initial psychiatric evaluation is used to focus on assessment of aspects of the patient's medical health, there could be less time available to address other issues that are of importance to the patient or of relevance to diagnosis and treatment planning.

Implementation

As described in the definition of "assessment" (see Glossary of Terms), there are a variety of ways clinicians may obtain recommended information about a patient's medical health during an initial psychiatric evaluation. Typically, an evaluation involves a direct interview between the patient and the clinician. In some circumstances (e.g., an evaluation of a patient with severe psychosis or dementia), obtaining information on history and a review of symptoms may not be possible through direct questioning. When available, prior medical records, electronic prescription databases, input from other treating clinicians, and information from family members or friends can raise previously unknown information. Added details or corroboration of information obtained in the interview is often helpful, since gaps in patient report can arise from ordinary errors in comprehension, recall, and expression (Redelmeier et al. 2001; Ryan et al. 2013; Simon et al. 2012). Flexibility may be needed in framing questions in terms that patients or family members are able to understand. For example, patients with intellectual disability or neurocognitive disorders may have difficulty in understanding questions as initially posed. In older individuals, difficulty understanding questions may signal unrecognized impairments in hearing or in cognition that would benefit from more detailed evaluation.

In some clinical contexts, such as a planned outpatient assessment, patients may be asked to complete an electronic- or paper-based form that inquires about key elements of the medical history and review of systems. Such forms may be completed prior to the visit or upon arrival at the office and can serve as a starting point to explore reported symptoms or historical information. Discussion may also be initiated with a brief open-ended question, which is conducive to capturing the nuances and narrative of the patient's concerns. Thus, with the sexual history, a patient may be asked "Do you have any sexual concerns or problems that you would like to discuss?" or "Are you sexually active?" (Althof et al. 2013), with follow-up questions asked (e.g., about contraceptive use), as indicated. Laboratory data or findings of electrocardiography, imaging studies, other radiological investigations or neuropsychological testing may also provide clues to past or current medical conditions.

These recommendations should not be viewed as representing a comprehensive set of questions relating to assessment of medical health, nor should they be seen as an endorsement of a checklist approach to evaluation. For example, there are frequent overlaps between medical health and substance use disorders, but recommendations for substance use assessment are provided in "Substance Use Assessment." Depending on the clinical setting and type of treatment, some information may be more or less relevant to obtain as part of the evaluation. Thus, it may be important to assess diseases and symptoms of disease that have a high prevalence among individuals with the patient's demographic characteristics and background, such as infectious disease in a patient who uses intravenous drugs or pulmonary and cardiovascular disease in a patient who smokes. Identifying a family history of hyperlipidemia or early cardiac death would be more relevant to obtain in an individual with multiple cardiac risk factors or a risk for metabolic syndrome. A detailed review of systems may be less crucial in a generally healthy individual who receives regular primary preventive care, although the Current Procedural Terminology and the U.S. Centers for Medicare and Medicaid Services describe the review of systems as a part of a comprehensive evaluation (Centers for

Medicare and Medicaid Services 2014; Schmidt et al. 2010). In patients who will be treated with psychotherapy by the psychiatrist who is performing the evaluation, some aspects of the history (e.g., sexual and reproductive history) may be more appropriate to defer until later in treatment.

Information may also be more or less relevant to obtain based on the timing of a clinical event. Time-based terms such as "current," "recent," or "past" are often used in clinical contexts but are impossible to define precisely and introduce vagueness into recommendations. With some information (e.g., allergies), details are essential to obtain regardless of when the clinical event may have occurred. With other information (e.g., minor surgical procedures, minor trauma), more recent events may be of relevance, whereas events in the distant past would be of minimal importance to elicit in a thorough fashion.

To determine whether the patient has an ongoing relationship with a primary care health professional requires gathering additional information besides a simple recording of the clinician's name. Some patients may be assigned to a primary care health professional, yet rarely meet with the individual or receive preventive care. Under such circumstances, inquiring about the patient's relationship with his or her primary care practitioner can be a starting point for improved access to quality health care and preventive services. For individuals who are receiving care from multiple specialty physicians, initial questions about having a primary care health professional can be followed up with additional questions about other clinicians who are providing them with care. Obtaining a complete and accurate list of the patient's medications can be challenging but has many implications for diagnosis and avoiding medication errors. When asked about the medications that they are taking, most patients think in terms of prescriptions they receive at a pharmacy, but they may not report receiving long-acting injectable antipsychotic medications, oral or long-acting injectable contraceptives, or non-prescribed medications (e.g., over-the-counter medications, vitamins, herbal products, nutritional supplements) unless specifically asked. Approaches that have been employed to develop an accurate medication list include using a structured format for the medication history (Drenth-van Maanen et al. 2011) or involving hospital-based clinical pharmacists or pharmacy technicians in taking a medication history (Brownlie et al. 2014; Kwan et al. 2013). With the use of electronic prescribing and electronic health records, information on patients' previous medications will be increasingly available to clinicians. Again, these data can be used as a starting point for discussion but still require verification by the clinician to ensure that the electronic information is correct and consistent with the patient's current use of the medication and pattern of adherence. Particularly with older individuals, it can be useful to remind patients to bring a current list of their medications and bring all of their medication bottles from home at the time of the visit. If a patient's recall of medications is inconsistent or erroneous, it may signal a need for detailed cognitive examination to identify possible neurocognitive impairments that would pose medication safety risks or interfere with adherence.

The physical examination may be performed by the psychiatrist, another physician, or a medically trained clinician. Elements of the examination, such as vital signs, height, and weight, may also be obtained by nursing staff or a medical assistant. The results of the patient's most recent physical examination may also be relied on in obtaining information about the patient's physical status. Considerations influencing the decision of whether the psychiatrist will personally perform the physical examination include potential effects on the psychiatrist-patient relationship, the purposes of the evaluation, and the complexity of the medical condition of the patient. The timing and scope of the examination will vary according to clinical circumstances. In some individuals, portions of the examination (e.g., vital signs) may be important to perform as soon as possible to identify an urgent need for referral (e.g., in a patient with symptoms of alcohol withdrawal). In other individuals, it may be appropriate to defer the examination. For example, the physical examination of an otherwise healthy patient with paranoia may be deferred to a different clinician or a more appropriate time or setting. Depending on the setting and type of treatment, transference issues could arise and interfere with effective treatment if the psychiatrist conducts the physical examination himself or herself. If physical assessments are done as part of the evaluation rather than relying on examinations by other health professionals, provisions for chaperones should be considered.

Barriers to the use of these recommendations also exist, with a major barrier being constraints on clinician time and the need to assess many aspects of the patient's symptoms and history within a circumscribed period. Depending on the setting, general health status, and other clinical characteristics of the patient, clinicians may judge other parts of the evaluation as having a greater priority in planning initial treatment. In terms of conducting a physical examination, assessment of some organ systems may be viewed as being outside the scope of typical psychiatric practice. In addition, many psychiatrists, particularly in an outpatient setting, will not have access to a fully equipped room for conducting physical examinations. For medically ill patients, elements of the physical examination, such as gait, may not be possible to assess because of the severity of the patient's condition. In other individuals, the severity of their psychiatric illness may limit their ability to collaborate with a general medical history, medication history, review of systems, and physical examination.

GUIDELINE VII. Quantitative Assessment

Guideline Statements

APA suggests (2C) that the initial psychiatric evaluation of a patient include quantitative measures of symptoms, level of functioning, and quality of life.

Rationale

The goal of this guideline is to improve, during and after an initial psychiatric evaluation, clinical decision making and treatment outcomes.

The strength of supporting research evidence for this guideline statement is low. Two studies were identified that compared the use of a quantitative measure with clinical interview in patients who presented with a psychiatric symptom, sign, or syndrome and that looked for an impact on clinical decision making. Both studies were observational in design, and both examined the use of a scale that assessed only for delirium. Use of the scale was associated with greater diagnostic accuracy as compared with assessment without the scale, but the effect was weak and the study population was limited to patients in an intensive care setting.

Many studies have addressed the development, use, and statistical characteristics of psychiatric rating scales, but there have not been specific comparisons of these measures and nonquantitative assessment. In addition, there has not been specific examination of effects on clinical decision making. Nevertheless, other studies have examined potential benefits and utility of quantitative measures in psychiatric practice and contribute to the rationale for using ratings scales in clinical practice. For example, in addition to use of the self-rated 9-item Patient Health Questionnaire (PHQ-9) in depression screening, benefits have been found when the PHQ-9 is used for ongoing monitoring of depressed patients, either by psychiatrists (Arbuckle et al. 2013; Chung et al. 2013; Duffy et al. 2008; Katzelnick et al. 2011) or in primary care settings (Yeung et al. 2012). The Sequenced Treatment Alternatives to Relieve Depression (STAR*D) study (Trivedi 2009; Trivedi et al. 2007) and other studies (Allen et al. 2009; Bickman et al. 2011; Zimmerman and McGlinchey 2008a; Zimmerman et al. 2011; Zubkoff et al. 2012) have shown success in the clinical implementation of quantitative measures and in the use of measurement-based approaches to clinical decision-making (i.e., "measurement-based care"). An additional study that randomly assigned patients to monthly use of standardized measures compared with treatment as usual showed a reduction in inpatient days, although subjective outcomes were unaffected (Slade et al. 2006). In studies of psychotherapy, systematic rating scales have been used to provide "outcome-informed treatment" in which patients provide feedback on levels of distress as well as on facets of the therapeutic alliance and perceived benefits of treatment (Boswell et al. 2015).

The field trials for DSM-5 also demonstrated the feasibility and reliability of using the DSM-5 Level 1 Cross-Cutting Symptom Measure in clinical practice (Narrow et al. 2013). Furthermore, research studies have demonstrated the validity and reliability of many quantitative measures, including both self- and clinician-administered scales, which can also be useful in routine clinical practice (Rush et al. 2008).

Despite insufficient research evidence, many experts agree that clinical decision making is improved by the use of quantitative measures in an initial psychiatric evaluation. Intuitively, and by analogy with other medical specialties in which standardized measurement (e.g., of physiological signs or laboratory tests) guides treatment, the use of a systematic and quantifiable approach to assessment would seemingly produce better patient outcomes and greater standardization of care across patients (Harding et al. 2011). Other experts contend that the benefits are uncertain or depend on clinical factors such as the setting of the evaluation and individual patient characteristics. Furthermore, expert opinion suggests that quantitative measures may not have clear advantages to a comprehensive interview by an experienced clinician and may even have disadvantages, such as inflexibility and cost, that are not clearly outweighed by the burden of using measures. These differences of opinion are reflected in the results of a survey of experts conducted by the APA, as described under "Review of Supporting Research Evidence."

Potential Benefits and Harms

Clinical decision making, including but not limited to diagnosis and treatment planning, requires a careful and systematic assessment of the type, frequency, and magnitude of psychiatric symptoms as well as an assessment of the impact of those symptoms on the patient's day-to-day functioning and quality of life. There are a number of potential benefits to obtaining this information as part of the initial psychiatric evaluation through the use of quantitative measures. Compared with a clinical interview, quantitative measures may help the clinician to conduct a more consistent and comprehensive review of the multiplicity of symptoms that the patient may be experiencing. This more comprehensive review may prevent the patient and the clinician from overlooking symptoms that are of potential relevance to diagnosis, treatment planning, and other clinical decision making. For example, subthreshold symptoms or comorbid subsyndromal conditions may be identified that are relevant to treatment planning and functioning. Similarly, the use of quantitative measures to assess the patient's level of functioning and quality of life may provide information about how illness affects the patient's daily life that is more consistent and comprehensive than information gained by clinical interview. Measures of the patient's level of functioning and quality of life may also signal the need for psychiatric or psychosocial interventions that target specific aspects of disability. If co-occurring medical illnesses are affecting level of functioning and quality of life, this may signal a need for consulting and collaborating with other treating clinicians or strengthening the patient's ability to cope with a chronic medical condition. Using systematic measures may also increase the efficiency of asking routine questions and allow more time for clinicians to focus on symptoms of greatest severity or issues of most concern to the patient.

Another key potential benefit of obtaining quantitative measures during an initial evaluation is to establish baseline measurements against which progress can be measured as treatment unfolds. For example, baseline data may help the clinician later to assess the adequacy of treatment or the need for treatment modifications as well as to interpret symptoms that emerge during the course of treatment, either related to progression of underlying psychiatric disorders or as side effects of treatments. Without the use of a consistent quantitative measure, recall biases may confound the ability of patients and clinicians to compare past and current levels or patterns of symptoms and functioning. When patients have had substantial improvements in symptoms and functioning, it can be easy to focus on the improvements and overlook residual symptoms or side effects of treatment that are contributing to ongoing impairment or quality of life. Ongoing use of quantitative assessments may also foster identification of residual symptoms or impairments and early detection of illness recurrence. Systematic use of quantitative measures can also facilitate communication among treating clinicians and can serve as a basis for enhanced management of populations of patients as well as individual patients.

Most patients will be able to appreciate the ways in which the use of quantitative measures will be of benefit to them. The fact that the clinician is using a systematic approach to address the patients' symptoms and functioning sends a positive message that could improve the therapeutic relationship. Especially in developed countries, patients are used to and expect digital, computerized information exchange, including for health-related monitoring and communication. For these patients, the use of quantitative measures within the context of an electronic health record, mobile app, or other computerized technology may have positive effects on the relationship of the patient with the psychiatrist and the health system.

Use of quantitative measures can have a number of potential harms. Overreliance on quantitative measures may lead other key elements of the patient's symptoms and life circumstances to be overlooked. Some patients may view quantitative measures as impersonal or may feel annoyed by having to complete detailed scales, particularly if done frequently. If a patient feels negatively about quantitative measures, this could alter the developing therapeutic alliance.

The amount of time available for an initial psychiatric evaluation is typically constrained by clinician availability, cost, and other factors. Under such circumstances, time that is used to obtain quantitative measures could introduce harms by reducing time available to address other issues of importance to the patient or of relevance to clinical decision making. Logistical barriers to using quantitative measures appear to be common. Depending on the patient characteristics, the setting, and the model of payment, using systematic ratings can be associated with financial costs. Systematic use of measures may require changes in workflow to distribute scales and additional time to review the results with the patient. Unreimbursed costs of practice may also increase if additional staff are needed to support modified workflows, if changes are needed to an electronic health record system to permit integration of measures, or if payment is needed to use copyrighted versions of scales.

Implementation

The specific tasks required for implementation of quantitative measurement will vary with the setting and the patient population served by the clinician's practice. In all situations, a necessary first step will be selecting appropriate scales for use. Selected measures should be appropriate for the clinical setting and should consider factors such as patient language, literacy, and health literacy. Other factors that can affect the statistical reliability and validity of rating scale measures include comorbid illnesses, race, ethnicity, and cultural background. It is important to consider whether the chosen scales have appropriate norms based on patient characteristics and setting. Depending on predictive values, sensitivity, and specificity, some rating scales may be better suited to screening whereas other rating scales may be better suited for detailed assessments of symptoms and for outcome monitoring. If more than one quantitative measure is being used, it is important to minimize duplication of questions and avoid overwhelming the patient with an excessive number of scales to complete. Rating scales should always be used as a supplement and not a replacement for clinical assessment and should be implemented in a way that supports development of the therapeutic relationship with the patient.

For assessment of psychiatric symptoms and behaviors across a range of domains, the DSM-5 Level 1 Cross-Cutting Symptom Measure (American Psychiatric Association 2013b) may be useful (Narrow et al. 2013). A self-report measure is available for adults and for children ages 11–17. A parent/guardian measure exists for children ages 6–17. Online versions of the measure are available at http://www.psychiatry.org/practice/dsm/dsm5/online-assessment-measures#Level1. Findings of the Level 1 measure can be amplified by follow-up questioning or by the use of additional measures, such as the DSM-5 Level 2 Cross-Cutting Symptom Measures. The My Mood Monitor (M-3) checklist (http://www.annfammed.org/content/suppl/2010/03/04/8.2.160.DC1/Gaynes_Supp_App.pdf; http://www.whatsmym3.com) is another self-report measure that screens for multiple disorders, including questions on depressive, bipolar, anxiety, obsessive-compulsive, and trauma-related disorders. Other specific rating scales may also be of use. For example, a number of clinician-rated and/

or self-rated scales have been widely used in research and are increasingly used in ongoing clinical monitoring of depression (Chung et al. 2013; Duffy et al. 2008; Katzelnick et al. 2011). These include the PHQ-9 (http://www.integration.samhsa.gov/images/res/PHQ%20-%20Questions.pdf; Kroenke et al. 2001), the clinician-rated Hamilton Rating Scale for Depression (Ham-D; http://health-net.umassmed.edu/mhealth/HAMD.pdf; Hamilton 1960; McIntyre et al. 2005), and the Inventory of Depressive Symptomatology (IDS), which is available in clinician-rated and self-rated versions (http://www.ids-qids.org/; Rush et al. 1996). Other symptom scales are described in *Handbook of Psychiatric Measures,* 2nd Edition, edited by Rush et al. (2008). For the assessment of functional impairments, the World Health Organization Disability Assessment Schedule 2.0 (WHODAS 2.0) is a 36-item, self-administered scale that also has a proxy-administered version (http://www.psychiatry.org/File%20Library/Practice/DSM/DSM-5/WHODAS2SelfAdministered.pdf; World Health Organization 2010). Quality of life can also be measured using a scale developed by the World Health Organization, the WHOQOL-BREF (http://depts.washington.edu/seaqol/WHOQOL-BREF; Skevington et al. 2004; The WHOQOL Group 1998). The Centers for Disease Control and Prevention (CDC) Healthy Days Measure (HRQOL-14) and core module (HRQOL-4) (http://www.cdc.gov/hrqol/hrqol14_measure.htm) have also been used in general population samples to assess physical and emotional symptoms as related to an individual's perceived sense of well-being (Moriarty et al. 2003). The Satisfaction With Life Scale (Diener et al. 1985; http://internal.psychology.illinois.edu/~ediener/SWLS.html) has been developed and used to assess life satisfaction and quality of life in individuals with chronic mental illness. For a nonspecific measure of quality of life, patients can be asked to rate their overall (physical and mental) quality of life in the past month on a scale from 0 ("about as bad as dying") to 10 ("life is perfect") (Unützer et al. 2002).

In some clinical contexts, such as a planned outpatient assessment, patients may be asked to complete electronic- or paper-based quantitative measures, either prior to the visit or upon arrival at the office (Allen et al. 2009; Harding et al. 2011; Trivedi 2009; Trivedi et al. 2007). Between or prior to visits, mobile technology may also be adaptable to obtaining quantitative measurements (Palmier-Claus et al. 2012). In other clinical contexts, such as acute inpatient settings, electronic modes of data capture may be more cumbersome and patients may need more assistance in completion of scales. As an alternative, proxy-based scales or clinician-rated scales may be used. Additional implementation considerations will depend on whether an electronic health record or other technologies are used within the practice. Some electronic health records may include built-in measurement functionality (e.g., default forms for rating of symptoms, functioning, or quality of life). As electronic health records become more commonly used, electronic capture of quantitative measures can allow computerized decision-support systems to be used in guiding evidence-based treatment (Trivedi et al. 2004), thereby improving outcomes and quality of care.

A number of barriers to implementing quantitative measures in routine clinical practice have been described (Harding et al. 2011; Valenstein et al. 2009; Zimmerman and McGlinchey 2008b; Zimmerman et al. 2011). Patient-related barriers include problems in completing scales because of psychiatric symptom severity, low health literacy, or reading difficulties. Some individuals may be unwilling to complete quantitative measures, although available information suggests that ambulatory patients are generally cooperative (Duffy et al. 2008; Narrow et al. 2013; Zimmerman and McGlinchey 2008a).

Quantitative measures themselves present additional barriers to implementation. Most scales have been developed and used primarily in research settings, and this can limit their generalizability, usability, and perhaps their reliability and validity in routine clinical use. There is limited consensus on the best measures to implement. Normative values are not always available, and it is even more uncommon to have normative values available based on factors such as educational level, age, race, ethnicity, culture, or comorbid conditions that can influence ratings. Variations in patient's health literacy, reading ability, and symptom severity can also lead patients to misinterpret questions. Other patients may bias the ratings that they record, either unintentionally (e.g., to please the clinician with their progress) or intentionally (e.g., to obtain controlled substances, to support claims of disability). Thus, the answers to questions and the summative scores on quantitative measures need to be interpreted in the context of the clinical presentation. Relying on a summative score can also be misleading when an overall scale score may be low but an important rating (e.g., suicidal ideas) is noted to be severe or frequent. Because many scales ask the patient to rate symptoms over several weeks, they may not be sensitive to change. This can be problematic in acute care settings, where treatment adjustments and symptom improvement can occur fairly quickly. Some symptom-based quantitative measures focus either on symptom frequency over the observation period or on symptom severity. Although these features often increase or decrease in parallel, that is not invariably the case. Other quantitative measures ask the patient to consider both symptom frequency and severity, which can also make the findings difficult to interpret.

Finally, as described under "Potential Benefits and Harms," cost may be a decisive barrier to the implementation of quantitative measures in usual clinical practice, particularly if the potential benefits are uncertain for the patients treated within a specific clinical practice. Costs may include time and resources needed to implement and administer measures (Harding et al. 2011; Veerbeek et al. 2012), including within existing electronic health records, as well as costs associated with obtaining permission or a license to use measures that are protected by copyright laws.

GUIDELINE VIII. Involvement of the Patient in Treatment Decision Making

Guideline Statements

Statement 1. APA recommends (1C) that the initial psychiatric evaluation of a patient who is seen include an explanation to the patient of the following: the differential diagnosis, risks of untreated illness, treatment options, and benefits and risks of treatment.
Statement 2. APA recommends that the initial psychiatric evaluation of a patient who is seen include asking the patient about treatment-related preferences.
Statement 3. APA recommends that the initial psychiatric evaluation of a patient who is seen include collaboration between the clinician and the patient about decisions pertinent to treatment.

Rationale

The goal of this guideline is to improve patient engagement, patient knowledge of diagnosis and treatment options, and collaborative decision making between patients and clinicians about treatment-related decisions.

The strength of research evidence supporting the educational and collaborative approaches recommended in statements 1, 2, and 3 is low. A number of randomized, controlled trials have studied the utility of similar approaches in the evaluation and treatment of individuals with a psychiatric disorder. However, as described in "Review of Supporting Research Evidence," the majority of the studies were nonblinded and had many potential confounding factors, and the applicability of the studies for this guideline is limited (e.g., because they studied individuals in a single setting or with a single diagnosis). Furthermore, the findings of these studies were weak and inconsistent. The positive studies demonstrated effects that were brief or small in magnitude. Positive outcomes were also indirectly related to treatment outcomes. For example, when patients were educated about their illness or treatment, measurements showed that their knowledge increased. Patient satisfaction tended to improve when information was conveyed through increased contact with the treatment team, but this was not necessarily the case when information was conveyed by printed materials only. Findings of studies on incorporating patient choices and on involving the patient in treatment decision making were mixed in terms of improved treatment adherence and clinical outcomes, respectively. Notably, however, studies did not demonstrate any harms of the interventions.

A number of investigators have examined treatment outcomes in relation to the patient's previously stated preferences. Studies have been conducted in psychiatric and in primary care settings in individuals with major depressive disorder or chronic forms of depression. Interventions have included antidepressant medication as compared with forms of psychotherapy (e.g., cognitive-behavioral therapy, cognitive behavioral analysis system of psychotherapy, supportive therapy) or combined treatment with antidepressant and psychotherapy. Findings of these studies are mixed, with some (Kocsis et al. 2009; Lin et al. 2005; Mergl et al. 2011) but not all (Dunlop et al. 2012; Kwan et al. 2010; Leykin et al. 2007; Steidtmann et al. 2012) showing greater or more rapid symptom reduction among individuals who received their preferred treatment. Other secondary analyses showed better reported therapeutic alliance among individuals who received their preferred treatment in some studies (Iacoviello et al. 2007; Kwan et al. 2010). Despite the variability of these results, these studies provide some indirect evidence that asking about patient preferences could influence the therapeutic alliance, adherence, or outcomes, at least in individuals with depression (Gelhorn et al. 2011).

Other indirect evidence for benefit comes from limited findings of improvements with medical and surgical patients' knowledge related to use of personalized risk communications (Edwards et al. 2013) or decision aids (Knops et al. 2013). Decisional conflict also shows some reductions related to use of decision aids (Stacey et al. 2011).

Despite this lack of strong supporting research evidence, experts agree that including the approaches recommended in statements 1, 2, and 3 as part of the initial psychiatric evaluation has benefits for enhancing the therapeutic alliance, treatment adherence, and patient and clinician satisfaction, and these potential benefits clearly outweigh the few potential harms.

These guideline statements are consistent with recommendations of the Institute of Medicine that patient-centered care be delivered as one element of high-quality health care (National Research Council 2001). Other organizations have promoted similar educational and collaborative approaches to care, often using the term "shared decision-making." For example, the U.S. Preventative Services Task Force has described how shared decision making may be incorporated into the delivery of preventative care (Sheridan et al. 2004). Shared decision making and informed patient choice have also been described as principles for the ethical practice of medicine (Drake and Deegan 2009; Moulton and King 2010). In particular, the ethical principles of respect for persons (National Commission for the Protection of Human Subjects of Biomedical and Behavioral Research 1979) and for autonomy (Beauchamp and Childress 2012) are well established and provide clear support for involvement of the patient. Involvement of the patient in decisions about his or her care is also an integral part of the ethical and legal tenets of informed consent (AMA Council on Ethical and Judicial Affairs 2012; Beauchamp 2011). Opinion 8.08 of the *Code of Medical Ethics of the American Medical Association* (AMA Council on Ethical and Judicial Affairs 2012) provides further discussion of informed consent including the need to "sensitively and respectfully disclose all relevant medical information to patients" in a manner so that the "quantity and specificity of this information [are] tailored to meet the preferences and needs of individual patients."

Potential Benefits and Harms

There are a number of potential benefits to discussing differential diagnosis, risks of untreated illness, treatment options, and benefits and risks of treatment with the patient at the time of an initial psychiatric evaluation. These include strengthening the therapeutic alliance and enhancing the patient's satisfaction with the care received, by respecting the patient's autonomy. Adherence may also be improved if the patient understands the reasoning behind a particular treatment approach. If an effective treatment is provided, improved adherence could be expected to be associated with reduced symptoms and improved functioning. The safety of treatment may also be enhanced if patients are educated about potential side effects of treatment, because knowledge about these potential effects could facilitate earlier reporting of difficulties with treatment.

Obtaining information about the patient's treatment-related preferences may also contribute to improved adherence, a stronger therapeutic alliance, and greater satisfaction with care. Because such preferences may have arisen from personal or family experiences with a specific treatment, they may provide clues to a patient's therapeutic or adverse responses to a given treatment or mechanistically similar treatments. Thus, an additional benefit of eliciting patient preferences may relate to the efficacy or safety of treatment for the individual patient.

Collaborating with the patient about decisions pertinent to treatment also has the potential to improve the therapeutic alliance, satisfaction with care, and adherence with treatment. Such collaboration may also increase the likelihood that the patient's expressed preferences will be integrated into the treatment plan.

Potential harms of these recommendations are minimal. It is possible that some individuals will not be interested in receiving information on differential diagnosis, risks of untreated illness, treatment options, and benefits and risks of treatment. Patients may also prefer not to be involved in collaborative decision making, feeling that the clinician is more knowledgeable or that the options are too overwhelming to consider.

It is difficult to estimate the cost of explaining the patient's differential diagnosis, risks of untreated illness, treatment options, and benefits and risks of treatment as well as inquiring about the patient's treatment-related preferences and collaborating with the patient in making decisions pertinent to treatment. The time required for each of these steps will differ with the patient and the clinical context. Such costs are also difficult to disentangle from the overall cost of an initial psychiatric evaluation. When factors including cost or model of payment constrain the amount of time available for an initial psychiatric evaluation, time that is used to focus on shared decision making could reduce time available to address other issues of importance to the patient or of relevance to diagnosis and treatment planning.

Implementation

These guideline recommendations apply to patients who have decision-making capacity. In general, individuals are presumed to have capacity unless there is compelling evidence to the contrary (Appelbaum 2007; Sessums et al. 2011). Capacity is presumed even in individuals who may have been admitted to a facility on an involuntary basis. Accordingly, the initial steps of a shared decision-making process are recommended for new patients, unless it is clear that the individual has severe cognitive impairment or disorganized thought processes that would impede his or her ability to process information. Even when disorganized thinking, delirium, or neurocognitive disorders are present, patients may still be able to understand some degree of information about their illness and its treatment and may be able to express some opinions about preferences. In individuals with delirium, such discussions may be able to occur during periods of greater lucidity. Initial steps to shared decision making include discussing the differential diagnosis, risks of untreated illness, treatment options, and benefits and risks of treatment. To assess the patient's knowledge after this information is conveyed, it is often useful to ask for a summary of his or her understanding of the diagnosis and treatment options. Assessing the patient's ability to understand this information is one element of assessing decision-making capacity (Appelbaum 2007). If the patient does not seem to fully grasp the information that was conveyed, the clinician will want to determine whether this reflects a true inability to understand the material or whether the explanation needs to be worded in more straightforward terms (Epstein and Gramling 2013; Epstein and Peters 2009; Sessums et al. 2011; Sheridan et al. 2004). Shifting to a different mode or format of presentation may also help improve the patient's understanding of the material (Covey 2007). With such adaptations, individuals with low health literacy, learning disabilities, or some cognitive impairment may still be able to learn key material and collaborate in their care. More detailed assessment for possible delirium or neurocognitive disorder is warranted if the patient has difficulty understanding the material when presented in a simpler format. With permission from the patient, the patient's family may also be involved to help the patient to understand treatment options and collaborate in care. In addition to determining whether the patient understands factual elements of the information that has been conveyed, it is also useful to inquire about any concerns, fears, preconceptions, or other beliefs that the patient has about the information. This can help in addressing miscommunications or in providing the patient with additional support if the fears or concerns are realistic.

A second element of assessing capacity is determining whether the patient can appreciate his or her condition and the likely outcomes of the possible treatment options. Some individuals may be able to understand key information but lack insight and ability to appreciate that a psychiatric condition is present (Appelbaum 2007; Owen et al. 2013). Other individuals may have unrecognized cognitive impairment that results in poor adherence or unwillingness to consider treatment. Still other individuals have delusions that compromise their ability to appreciate the true consequences of an intervention (e.g., medication is believed to be poisonous, imaging studies are believed to be capable of activating embedded transmitters).

Asking patients about treatment-related preferences provides information about the outcomes that are most important to them. Desired outcomes may be broad in scope and encompass social and functional outcomes as well as symptomatic outcomes (Deegan and Drake 2006; Klein et al. 2007). Inquiring about the patient's current quality of life and level of functioning can often serve as a starting point for discussing his or her overarching goals and preferences for achieving them. For some individuals, avoiding a specific side effect may be more important than a difference in possible benefits. For other individuals, preferences may relate to pragmatic issues such as medication or treatment costs or availability of transportation for follow-up visits. As another aspect of patient preference, it is helpful to ask whether or not the patient wishes to have family members or others (e.g., case managers, close friends) involved in discussions or decisions about aspects of care including treatment. The majority of individuals want family involvement, although there is significant heterogeneity in the extent and type of involvement that is desired (Cohen et al. 2013). Increasing numbers of young adults reside with their parents (Vespa et al. 2013), suggesting the need to explore with patients the ways in which family members can help them meet their identified treatment goals (Dixon et al. 2014). In discussing the patient's preferences and choice of treatment, the clinician will be able to determine whether the patient is able to reason about treatment options and communicate a choice about treatment, which are the remaining elements of an assessment of decision-making capacity (Appelbaum 2007). For the majority of individuals (who have decision-making capacity), the clinician will have communicated key information through this process and will have engaged the patient in a collaborative approach to care.

Given that shared decision making is intended to focus on and integrate the unique aspects of the patient's preferences and options for treatment (Makoul and Clayman 2006), some flexibility in implementing these recommendations will be essential. One proposed model of shared decision making emphasizes the respectful exploration of "what matters most" to the patient (Elwyn et al. 2012). The dynamic and iterative aspects of discussion and decision making are also useful to keep in mind (Elwyn et al. 2012; Makoul and Clayman 2006). Although the shared decision-making process is recommended to begin during the initial evaluation, it will also continue and evolve throughout the patient's therapeutic relationship with the clinician.

The exact content of discussions with the patient may also vary depending on the circumstances. For example, when obtaining and documenting informed consent for a procedure or treatment with significant risk, a greater level of detail will be needed that outlines the specific risk and benefits of the proposed treatment and other possible options, include no treatment. On the other hand, a detailed discussion of the risks of forgoing treatment may not be crucial in an individual who implicitly knows the problems with untreated illness and is actively seeking assistance. In other circumstances, a patient's symptoms may not fulfill criteria for a specific diagnosis, or a final diagnosis may require additional history or review of information. Nevertheless, it may still be appropriate to initiate treatment based on what is already established. The clinician could discuss the likely diagnostic possibilities or explain why symptomatic treatment is still indicated, even in the absence of a clear diagnosis. Other elements of the proposed treatment approach may also contain uncertainties (Epstein and Gramling 2013), and gaps in available evidence may not allow estimates of risks and benefits of treatment. Again, the goal is a straightforward discussion of the therapeutic options as well as transparent mention of key areas of uncertainty that would be relevant to the patient's preferences and decisions. If electronic decision aids are available and relevant to the patient, these can be helpful (Friedberg et al. 2013; Sheridan et al. 2004; Stacey et al. 2011).

Communications with patients about their goals may involve a series of conversations rather than a single discussion. Patients may have additional questions and may make additional decisions about their care as their illness, their understanding of their symptoms, and their treatment options evolve. Family members and others whom the patient chooses to involve in his or her care may also have questions that arise over the course of treatment. For patients who are being treated with a type of treatment (e.g., assertive community treatment) or in a setting (e.g., hospital) that has a multidisciplinary team approach to care, other team members play an important role in discussing information with patients and families, clarifying issues of concern or confusion, and providing information in a format and level of detail that is appropriate to the patient's needs. In some settings, the multidisciplinary team members will collaborate with the patient and involved family members in developing an individualized treatment plan.

When a patient lacks capacity or is experiencing acute symptoms (e.g., delusions, agitation) that compromise informed discussion, shared decision making may not be possible or may need to be implemented more gradually as the patient's symptoms remit. Opinions 8.081 and 8.082 of the Code of Medical Ethics of the American Medical Association (AMA Council on Ethical and Judicial Affairs 2012) discuss circumstances in which informed-consent discussions may need to be modified or delayed or in which surrogate consent may be needed. When individuals who lack capacity have a surrogate decision-maker, a similar process can be followed that incorporates explaining the diagnosis and treatment options, eliciting preferences, and collaborating in decisions about treatment.

Some individuals may have completed a psychiatric advance directive that provides information about their preferences with regard to medication or other interventions (Elbogen et al. 2007). Limited evidence suggests that such advance directives can improve patient adherence with treatment (Wilder et al. 2010). Individuals with cognitive impairment may also have developed an advance care plan that describes their future wishes (Dening et al. 2011; Robinson et al. 2012). Patients can be encouraged to consider completing a psychiatric advance directive, advance care plan, or health care proxy at a time when they have the decisional capacity to do so (Moye et al. 2013; Srebnik et al. 2004).

A number of barriers exist to implementing these recommendations. Not all patients are interested in learning detailed information about diagnosis or treatment, or they may not be psychologically able to process and come to terms with the information. Patients are not always comfortable with a shared decision-making approach. Some patients may be reluctant to engage in discussion and may be fearful of how they will be viewed by the clinician (Frosch et al. 2012). Studies of patients with medical or surgical conditions suggest that there is significant variability in patient preferences related to shared decision making (Chewning et al. 2012; Singh et al. 2010). Furthermore, these preferences can be difficult to judge (Kon 2012) and may be culturally mediated (Charles et al. 2006). They are not absolute but may shift with the clinical context or type of decision that is being made (Epstein and Gramling 2013). Fewer studies are available in psychiatric patients, but these also suggest individual variations in preferences (Deegan and Drake 2006; Klein et al. 2007; Woltmann and Whitley 2010). Even for patients who are well informed and have high health literacy, shared decision making can sometimes impose an unrealistic burden on patients (Olthuis et al. 2014).

Other barriers relate to the amount of time that the clinician has available to engage in shared decision making or the lack of other resources (e.g., reimbursement, decision aids, other health professional staff) to help support the shared decision-making process (Friedberg et al. 2013; Légaré and Witteman 2013; Légaré et al. 2008; Sheridan et al. 2004). Clinicians may also lack knowledge about how to implement shared decision making, question its utility, or have concerns that it will complicate the therapeutic relationship (Friedberg et al. 2013; Légaré and Witteman 2013; Légaré et al. 2008; Sheridan et al. 2004). Some clinicians may be accustomed to interacting with patients in a paternalistic or authoritarian manner, which can present a barrier to open communication about patient preferences and values (Frosch et al. 2012). Thus, changes may be needed in clinician training and in the resources devoted to shared decision making to promote the implementation of these recommendations.

GUIDELINE IX. Documentation of the Psychiatric Evaluation

Guideline Statements

Statement 1. APA recommends (1C) that the initial psychiatric evaluation of a patient include documentation of the rationale for treatment selection, including discussion of the specific factors that influenced the treatment choice.
Statement 2. APA suggests (2C) that the initial psychiatric evaluation of a patient include documentation of the rationale for clinical tests.

Rationale

The goal of this guideline is to improve clinical decision making and increase coordination of psychiatric treatment with other clinicians.

The strength of the research evidence supporting statements 1 and 2 is low. No prospective studies were identified that addressed whether decision making about a patient's psychiatric diagnosis and treatment plan or coordination of psychiatric treatment with other clinicians is improved when the clinician documents the rationale for treatment selection and for clinical tests. However, some indirect information suggests that such a practice may be beneficial.

With the increasing use of electronic record systems, the structured but fragmented information that is common in electronic record notes can increase cognitive workload and reduce the quality of communication among those caring for the patient (Cusack et al. 2013; Embi et al. 2013; Mamykina et al. 2012; Rosenbloom et al. 2011). A greater emphasis on synthesizing information through documentation may ameliorate some of those difficulties. Clinical decision making may also be enhanced. The thought process behind clinical decision making is frequently described as having two distinct components—one that is intuitive, relying primarily on pattern recognition and rules-of-thumb, and one that is more systematic and analytical (Bate et al. 2012; Croskerry et al. 2013). The intuitive process is faster but more likely to introduce cognitive biases and error than the more reflective process. Although documenting the rationale for treatment selection and testing in addition to the usual practice of documenting the differential diagnosis may require additional time to complete, it may also allow clinicians to avoid biases and errors in clinical judgment and think about whether other care approaches and testing strategies may be more concordant with evidence-based practices or with the patient's needs and preferences.

Potential Benefits and Harms

In an initial psychiatric evaluation, documenting the rationale for treatment selection and clinical tests is potentially beneficial in several respects. When a patient's care is being provided by multiple individuals using a shared treatment or treatment team approach, collaboration and coordination of care among involved health professionals are crucial. Delineating the reasons for selecting treatment(s) and obtaining clinical tests can enhance collaboration and minimize misunderstandings or errors in the delivered treatment. Whether a patient is being cared for by one clinician or by many, documentation of clinical reasoning can be informative to review if questions arise later in treatment or if treatment is transitioned to different clinicians.

The amount of time available for an initial psychiatric evaluation is typically constrained by clinician availability, cost, and other factors. Under such circumstances, focusing on more detailed documentation of clinical decision making could introduce harms by reducing time available to address other issues of importance to diagnosis, treatment planning, or the patient. The financial cost of documenting the rationale for treatment selection and clinical tests is difficult to disentangle from the overall cost of an initial psychiatric evaluation, which varies depending on the patient, the setting, and the model of payment.

Implementation

When the clinician is describing the rationale for treatment selection and for clinical tests as part of the initial psychiatric evaluation, the breadth and depth of documentation will depend on the clinical circumstances and complexity of the decision making. Although some treatment or testing decisions may seem "intuitively obvious" (e.g., prescribing an antidepressant to a patient with depression, obtaining "routine" laboratory tests), the rationale for deciding among available therapeutic options almost always includes additional nuances. Thus, it is important to discuss the factors that influenced the treatment choice, such as the target symptom or syndrome being addressed by the treatment, the patient's preferences regarding treatment, the potential side effects of treatment relative to other options, and the past responses of the patient to treatment (if applicable). If the evaluation is done at the request of another health professional (i.e., as a consultation), enough detail should be included to permit the requestor of the consultation to follow through with any recommended actions. More detailed consideration and documentation of the risks and benefits of treatment options may also be needed in the following circumstances: when the planned treatment is a relatively costly, nonstandard treatment approach (e.g., multiple antipsychotic medications, "off-label" use of a medication) or has a heightened risk (e.g., use of clozapine or monoamine oxidase inhibitors); when involved parties disagree about the optimal course of treatment; when the patient's motivation or capacity to benefit from potential treatment alternatives is in question; when the treatment would be involuntary or when other legal or administrative issues are involved; or when available treatment options are limited by external constraints (e.g., financial barriers, insurance restrictions, geographic barriers, service availability, the patient's capacity to participate in the proposed treatment). In situations where informed consent is being obtained, the rationale for the therapeutic decision making will typically include the elements of the informed-consent discussion (e.g., risks and benefits of treatment options, including reasonable alternatives to the planned treatment; the patient's understanding of and acceptance of the treatment plan). If interventions such as hospitalization are planned as a result of the evaluation, their rationale is important to include in the discussion. Although this recommendation is limited to the initial psychiatric evaluation, some clinicians find it helpful to document their reasons for starting or stopping treatments or contingency plans (e.g., to address side effects or nonresponse) at other patient encounters as well.

The decision to do laboratory studies and other clinical tests, such as imaging studies, electrocardiography (ECG), or electroencephalography (EEG), should be based on the likelihood that the test result will alter diagnostic or treatment-related decision making. The costs of "routine" testing, in financial terms and in unneeded evaluations for false positive results, are unlikely to offset the benefits of untargeted testing.

The documentation of the rationale for treatment and testing can be a natural outgrowth of a biopsychosocial formulation, or it can be recorded separately as part of the diagnostic impression and plan. The overarching goal of the documentation is to provide a concise synthesis of the clinical thought process that permits ready access to important information in a manner that is reliable and consistent with the patient's clinical picture and helps in anticipating the patient's needs. These elements of documentation have been suggested as characteristics of quality in electronic record documentation (Hammond et al. 2010) but are equally relevant to paper-based formats.

Clinicians should be aware that the recommendations for assessment and documentation described in this guideline may differ from those outlined as part of a comprehensive evaluation according to the Current Procedural Terminology and the U.S. Centers for Medicare and Medicaid Services (Centers for Medicare and Medicaid Services 2014; Schmidt et al. 2010).

Documentation of psychiatric evaluations in general and of the rationales for treatment and testing in particular should be sensitive to issues of confidentiality. Medical records may also be viewed by others in addition to the clinician writing the note or other members of an interdisciplinary treatment team. Individuals who may sometimes view documentation include the patient, third-party payers, quality assurance/peer review evaluators, and, in certain jurisdictions, the executor of an estate after a patient's death. Furthermore, records may be part of future or current legal or administrative hearings, including disability litigation, divorce and custody adjudication, competency determinations, and actions of medical licensing boards. Electronic record systems have many different approaches to controlling access to records, with some restricting access of psychiatric notes to a small circle of individuals to optimize patient privacy, and others allowing broader access to notes with the aim of integrating medical and psychiatric care. Such factors need to be taken into consideration when the clinician is documenting.

Although the additional time required for documentation can be an added cost, some practitioners find that transcription or voice recognition software is useful in reducing documentation times while still permitting the details of clinical decision making to be captured. With electronic record systems, the use of copy/paste can improve the continuity of treatment plan documentation from visit to visit, but it must be used cautiously, because copying and pasting of text can lead to inaccuracies in documentation.

Review of Available Evidence

GUIDELINE I. Review of Psychiatric Symptoms, Trauma History, and Psychiatric Treatment History

Clinical Question

Development of this guideline was premised on the following clinical question:

For patients present with a psychiatric symptom, sign, or syndrome in any setting, are accuracy of diagnosis and appropriateness of treatment selection improved when the initial psychiatric evaluation typically (i.e., almost always) includes review of the following?

- **Psychiatric systems, including mood, anxiety, thought content and process, perceptual and cognitive problems, and trauma history**
- **Previous psychiatric diagnoses (both principal and working)**
- **Past psychiatric treatment trials (type, duration, and, where applicable, doses)**
- **Adherence to past psychiatric treatments, including both pharmacological and nonpharmacological treatments**
- **Response to past psychiatric treatments**

Review of Supporting Research Evidence

Overview of Studies

There is no supporting research evidence that specifically addresses the clinical question above.

Grading of Quality of Individual Studies

Not applicable.

Grading of Supporting Body of Research Evidence

Not applicable.

Differences of Opinion in Rating the Strength of Recommendations

None.

Expert Opinion Data: Results

To what extent do you agree that accuracy of diagnosis and appropriateness of treatment selection are improved when the initial psychiatric evaluation of any patient typically (i.e., almost always) includes review of the following?

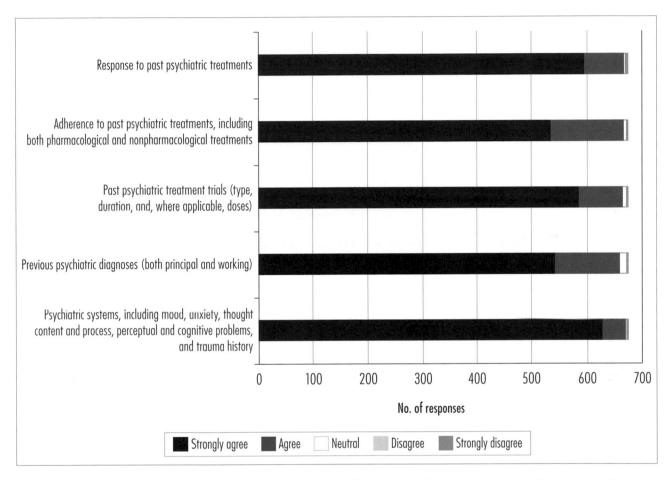

Percentage of experts who "strongly agreed" or "agreed" that accuracy of diagnosis and appropriateness of treatment selection is improved when the initial psychiatric evaluation of any patient typically (i.e., almost always) includes review of the following:

Response to past psychiatric treatments	99.1%
Adherence to past psychiatric treatments, including both pharmacological and nonpharmacological treatments	98.7%
Past psychiatric treatment trials (type, duration, and, where applicable, doses)	98.4%
Previous psychiatric diagnoses (both principal and working)	97.8%
Psychiatric systems, including mood, anxiety, thought content and process, perceptual and cognitive problems, and trauma history	99.3%

Do you typically (i.e., almost always) review these items during initial psychiatric evaluations of your patients?

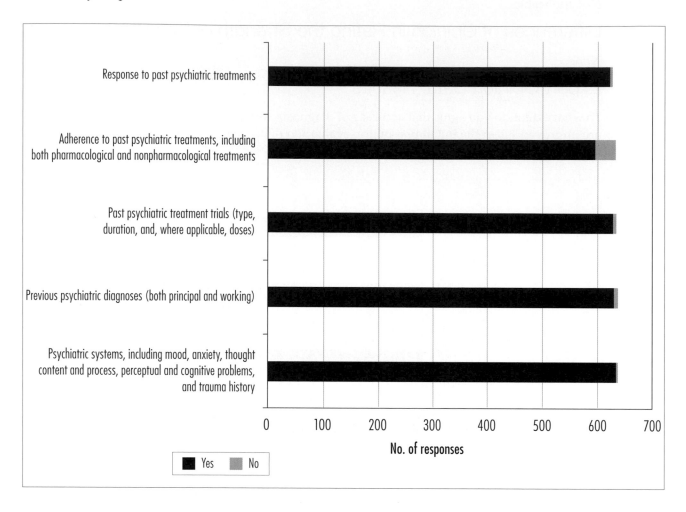

GUIDELINE II. Substance Use Assessment

Clinical Question

Development of this guideline was premised on the following clinical question:

For patients who present with a psychiatric symptom, sign, or syndrome in any setting, are identification and diagnosis of substance use disorders improved when the initial psychiatric evaluation typically (i.e., almost always) includes assessments of the following? 1) current tobacco use, 2) current alcohol use, 3) current use of other substances (e.g., marijuana, cocaine, heroin, psychomimetics), 4) current misuse of prescribed or over-the-counter (OTC) medications or supplements, 5) past tobacco use, 6) past alcohol use, 7) past use of other substances (e.g., marijuana, cocaine, heroin, psychomimetics), 8) past misuse of prescribed or OTC medications or supplements?

Review of Supporting Research Evidence

Overview of Studies

Study	Subjects/Method	N	Design/ Duration	Outcomes
Agabio et al. 2007	Patients with mood disorders treated in the outpatient clinic of the University of Cagliari, Italy, were asked to fill out alcohol-related questionnaires to determine the prevalence of alcohol use disorders and at-risk drinking, and to compare the sensitivity and specificity of the questionnaires.	56	Cross-sectional study design; subjects were recruited from May to November 2006.	Fourteen subjects (25%) met the criteria for alcohol use disorders according to the Structured Clinical Interview for DSM-IV (SCID-I); 17 (30.4%) achieved a score ≥ 1 on the CAGE questionnaire; 12 (21.4%) reached AUDIT scores of ≥ 8 and 4 for men and women, respectively; 12 (21.4%) provided positive answers to the National Institute on Alcohol Abuse and Alcoholism (NIAAA) Guide. Despite these prevalence rates, no diagnosis of alcohol use disorders had previously been registered in the medical records of the subjects who met SCID-I criteria for current alcohol use disorder. The CAGE questionnaire achieved the highest values of sensitivity and specificity in detecting alcohol use disorders tested against that of the SCID-I.
Hill and Chang 2007	Patients in a psychiatric outpatient clinic completed T-ACE (Tolerance, Annoyed, Cut down, Eye-opener), AUDIT, clinician interview, and SCID, to determine if the T-ACE and AUDIT improved identification of at-risk drinking.	50	Cross-sectional study design; subjects were recruited from January 2004 to February 2005.	Compared with the SCID, the sensitivities and specificities for T-ACE were 0.88 and 0.59, and those for AUDIT were 0.63 and 0.85. Brief screening instruments improved the identification of risky drinking at this psychiatry clinic.
Barry et al. 2006	Patients at a psychiatry emergency service were asked to complete an alcohol-related questionnaire to determine the prevalence of at-risk drinking. Patients with schizophrenia or bipolar disorder were compared with those with depression or anxiety.	390	Cross-sectional study design; subjects were recruited from 2001 to 2005.	Thirty-four patients (23%) with schizophrenia or bipolar disorder and 53 patients (22%) with depression or anxiety drank more than the recommended limits. Those with schizophrenia or bipolar disorder reported experiencing significantly more consequences from drinking than those with depression or anxiety.
Stasiewicz et al. 2008	Patients at a community mental health center with either schizophrenia spectrum or bipolar disorder and an alcohol use disorder were asked to complete assessments, including self-reports of recent alcohol use. This information was compared with collateral reports and with results of urine drug screens.	167	Cross-sectional study design; subjects were recruited within 2 weeks of treatment entry.	Overall, there was poor subject-collateral agreement, though better for subjects with negative urine drug screens ($n=97$). The most consistent predictor of subject-collateral discrepancy scores was subjects' recent drug use. This study emphasizes the need to enhance the validity of self-reports of substance use.

Grading of Quality of Individual Studies

Citation: Agabio R, Marras P, Gessa GL, Carpiniello B: Alcohol use disorders, and at-risk drinking in patients affected by a mood disorder, in Cagliari, Italy: sensitivity and specificity of different questionnaires. *Alcohol and Alcoholism* 42(6):575–581, 2007

Population: A nonstratified sample of 200 medical records was randomly selected (every third record) from among records of outpatients admitted to the Division of Psychiatry, University of Cagliari, for mood disorders from May to November 2006. Each patient was invited by phone to participate in the study; 56 patients participated.

Intervention: Patients were interviewed for about an hour and completed several alcohol-related questionnaires. Patients were informed about the size of a standard drink and then requested to answer questions of the first step of the NIAAA Guide, the AUDIT, and the CAGE ("Cut down," "Annoyed," "Guilty," Eye Opener") questionnaire. The SCID-I application forms for mood and alcohol disorders were also administered.

Outcomes: Fourteen subjects (25%) met the criteria for alcohol use disorders according to SCID-I; 17 (30.4%) achieved a score ≥1 on the CAGE questionnaire; 12 (21.4%) reached AUDIT scores of ≥8 and 4 for men and women, respectively; 12 (21.4%) provided positive answers to the NIAAA Guide questions. Despite these prevalence rates, no diagnosis of alcohol use disorders had previously been registered in the medical records of patients who met SCID-I criteria for current alcohol use disorders. The CAGE questionnaire achieved the highest values of sensitivity and specificity in detecting alcohol use disorders tested against that of the SCID-I.

Comparators: This study used a prior study (Grant et al. 2004) and meta-analysis (Sullivan et al. 2005) as comparator data.

Timing: The interview for each subject lasted about an hour. Data were collected from May to November 2006.

Setting: Outpatients from the Division of Psychiatry, University of Cagliari, Italy.

Study design: Cross-sectional.

Overall risk of study bias: **Moderate**

- **Selection bias:** *High Risk:* Not all patients who were asked agreed to be part of the study, and those who chose to participate may have had different drinking patterns from those who refused.
- **Performance bias:** *Low Risk:* There is no evidence of systematic differences in the treatment of participants or of protocol deviation.
- **Attrition bias:** *Low Risk:* Not applicable to this study because of the cross-sectional design. Data were collected once, with no follow-up.
- **Detection bias:** *High Risk:* Patients are likely to underreport their drinking when directly asked in questionnaires, and the in-person interview may have increased this likelihood. There was no effort to verify the information reported by the subjects.
- **Reporting bias:** *Low Risk:* Because an in-person interview was conducted, it is possible the interviewer recorded only information that fit within set parameters. However, because standardized, validated instruments were used, this risk is low.
- **Sponsor-related bias:** *Low Risk:* Article was published in a peer-reviewed journal with no obvious source of industry, institutional, or investigator bias.

Applicability: This study was performed in Italy in a mood disorder clinic and only addressed alcohol use. This may limit the generalizability of its findings to the United States, to individuals with other psychiatric diagnoses, and to individuals using other substances. Also, the assessment of drinking behavior was performed in a separate interview, rather than as part of the initial assessment, which may reduce applicability to the clinical question.

Citation: Hill KP, Chang G: Brief screening instruments for risky drinking in the outpatient psychiatry clinic. *American Journal of Addictions* **16(3):222–226, 2007**

Population: The Health and Habits Survey was given to 149 adult patients initiating psychiatric care in the psychiatric clinic of the Brigham and Women's Hospital in Boston, Massachusetts, between January 2004 and February 2005. These patients were invited to return on a separate visit to complete a SCID and the AUDIT; 50 patients agreed and were enrolled in the study. Ability to complete the Health and Habits Survey and willingness to participate in the study were the inclusion criteria.

Intervention: Patients were screened for alcohol use with the Health and Habits Survey, which contained questions about diet, smoking, exercise, stress, and usual drinking, and the T-ACE (Tolerance, Annoyed, Cut down, Eye-opener), a four-item alcohol screening instrument. Patients who agreed to enroll in the study completed a SCID and the AUDIT. All SCID interviews were administered by the same physician, who also obtained informed consent.

Comparators: Sensitivity and specificity of the T-ACE were compared with those of the AUDIT, using the SCID as a reference, for the 50 patients who went on to complete the AUDIT after the initial survey.

Outcomes: Brief screening instruments improved the identification of risky drinking in an outpatient psychiatry clinic compared with clinician interviews. The AUDIT identified risky drinking with a moderate sensitivity (0.63) and a high specificity (0.85). The T-ACE was less specific (0.59) but more sensitive (0.88) than the AUDIT.

Timing: Data were collected between January 2004 and February 2005. Potential subjects first completed the Health and Habits Survey and the T-ACE. Then, those who agreed to complete the SCID and the AUDIT returned at a later date, within a few weeks and as close as possible to the clinician intake interview.

Setting: Outpatient psychiatric clinic of Brigham and Women's Hospital, Boston, Massachusetts.

Study design: Cross-sectional.

Overall risk of study bias: **High**

- **Selection bias:** *High Risk:* Patients selected themselves for the study after learning about it. It is probable that those who consumed larger amounts of alcohol would be less likely to agree to participate in the study.
- **Performance bias:** High Risk: There was no blinding in this study; the clinician who performed the SCID was aware of the patients' T-ACE scores.
- **Attrition bias:** *High Risk:* Although the study defined enrolled subjects as the ones who completed the survey and then agreed to return to complete the SCID and the AUDIT, there is a potential for attrition bias in that only 50 of the initial 149 who completed the survey agreed to return. Those who chose not to proceed in the full study may have had different characteristics than those who did proceed.

- **Detection bias:** *High Risk:* Patients tend to underreport their drinking on surveys and interviews, and there was no attempt to verify information that was being given by self-report.
- **Reporting bias:** *Low Risk:* Since standardized instruments were used, and the same clinician was used for every SCID, the likelihood of reporting bias is low.
- **Sponsor-related bias:** *Low Risk:* This research was supported in part by grants from the American Psychiatric Institute for Research and Education and from the National Institute on Alcohol Abuse and Alcoholism, Bethesda, Maryland, as well as by the Dupont Warren Fellowship from Harvard Medical School, Boston, Massachusetts. There is no obvious source of bias from these sponsors.

Applicability: This study identified "risky drinking," which may or may not constitute an alcohol use disorder. Also, subjects were assessed outside of a standard psychiatric evaluation, which may limit the applicability of the study findings to the identification and diagnosis of substance use disorders as part of the initial psychiatric evaluation.

Citation: Barry KL, Milner K, Blow FC, et al.: Screening psychiatric emergency department patients with major mental illnesses for at-risk drinking. *Psychiatric Services* 57(7):1039–1042, 2006

Population: All eligible adult psychiatric emergency service patients age 18 years and older were asked to complete the informed consent form. Patients were excluded from the study if they were intoxicated, were incarcerated, had acute psychosis, were being seen for an overdose, had suicide attempts, had a legal guardian, or were too medically ill to participate. A total of 460 psychiatric emergency service patients were approached; 390 (80%) agreed to participate and completed questionnaires. An additional 214 patients did not meet inclusion criteria.

Intervention: Participants completed a questionnaire adapted from the Health Screening Survey, including quantity or frequency items for alcohol use, dieting, tobacco, and exercise in the previous 3 months; perceptions of a past or current alcohol problem; and seven past-year alcohol consequence items from the AUDIT.

Comparators: Analyses compared at-risk drinkers who had a serious mental illness (schizophrenia or bipolar disorder) with those who had depression or anxiety.

Outcomes: Thirty-four persons with schizophrenia or bipolar disorder (23%) and 53 with depression or anxiety (22%) drank heavily, according to NIAAA guidelines; engaged in binge drinking; reported a perception of a current problem with alcohol; or reported two or more alcohol-related consequences. Among the at-risk drinkers, the group with schizophrenia or bipolar disorder drank an average of 23.7±34.1 drinks per week; the group with depression or anxiety drank 24.3±27.8 drinks per week. There was a significant difference between the two diagnostic groups in use of any alcohol (62 persons with schizophrenia or bipolar disorder, or 42%, compared with 140 persons with depression or anxiety, or 58%). In the group with schizophrenia or bipolar disorder, 31 (91%) of the at-risk drinkers reported a past problem with alcohol, and 20 (59%) reported a current problem. In contrast, in the group with depression or anxiety, 34 (64%) of the at-risk drinkers reported a past problem, and 34 (64%) reported a current problem. Other differences were found between the patients with schizophrenia or bipolar disorder and those with depression or anxiety, including differences in education level and smoking status.

Timing: The study was conducted from 2001 to 2005.

Setting: Psychiatric emergency room in Ann Arbor, Michigan.

Study design: Cross-sectional.

Overall risk of study bias: **High**

- **Selection bias:** *High Risk:* There were several exclusion criteria involving medical illness, psychiatric symptoms, and legal status. These led to 214 people being excluded and 390 being included. Also, 20% of those approached for the study refused to participate, and the characteristics of those who refused may be different from those of the participants.
- **Performance bias:** *High Risk:* There was no blinding in this study, and so both participants and researchers knew who was in the study. Answers to questions may have been affected by knowledge of being in the study. The study compared different diagnostic groups (i.e., those with schizophrenia or bipolar disorder with those with depression or anxiety), and researchers knew participants' diagnoses
- **Attrition bias:** *Not applicable to this study* because there was no follow-up.
- **Detection bias:** *High Risk:* The study used a self-report questionnaire with no attempt to verify the information. Patients are likely to underreport drinking behavior in surveys that are based only on self-report. Additionally, the assessment included questions about past alcohol use, which participants answered by recall from memory.
- **Reporting bias:** *Low Risk:* There is no evidence of selective outcome reporting.
- **Sponsor-related bias:** *Low Risk:* The study was sponsored by the Flinn Family Foundation. There is no obvious source of bias from the investigators or the sponsor of this study.

Applicability: This study reported findings from a questionnaire given to psychiatric emergency patients, which may limit the applicability of this study to other clinical settings. The study also examined whether participants exhibited "at risk drinking," which may limit the applicability of the study in terms of identification and diagnosis of substance use disorders.

Citation: Stasiewicz PR, Vincent PC, Bradizza CM, et al.: Factors affecting agreement between severely mentally ill alcohol abusers' and collaterals' reports of alcohol and other substance abuse. *Psychology of Addictive Behaviors* **22(1):78–87, 2008**

Population: The subjects were 207 men and women seeking outpatient dual-diagnosis treatment from a university-affiliated community mental health center. Forty subjects (19%) were excluded from analyses because of missing baseline collateral data. Subjects were eligible if they had lived at their current address for at least 6 months or could provide two persons as locators; scored at least 23 (with scores of 22 considered on a case-by-case basis) on the Mini-Mental State Exam to ensure adequate cognitive functioning for study participation; and met DSM-IV criteria for a current (i.e., past 12 months) alcohol use disorder and a current schizophrenia spectrum or bipolar disorder.

Intervention: Subjects were recruited within 2 weeks of treatment entry and completed measures of cognitive functioning, alcohol dependence severity, psychiatric symptoms, and quantity and frequency of substance use over the previous 60 days using the Timeline Followback interview (Sobell et al. 1996). They also provided a urine sample, which was screened for recent substance use. Collateral interviews were conducted by phone and included an assessment of the subject's alcohol and substance use over the same 60-day period. Collaterals also reported their confidence in the accuracy of their reports.

Comparators: Subject reports of substance use were compared with reports from collateral interviews and with the results of urine toxicology screens. Collateral interview reports and urine toxicology screen results were also compared.

Outcomes: Overall, the results indicated generally poor subject-collateral agreement. Collateral report rarely provided more information on substance use than subject report, which as the authors noted, "calls into question the value of routine use of collateral informants." The most consistent predictor of subject-collateral discrepancy scores was subjects' recent drug use; subject-collateral agreement appeared better for those individuals with negative urine drug screens ($n=97$). In contrast, there was high agreement between subjects' self-report and results of the urine toxicology screen. Agreement was lower, though still in an acceptable range, between collateral report and urine toxicology screen results.

Timing: Subjects were recruited within 2 weeks of treatment entry. There were two study visits: a diagnostic interview to determine diagnosis and study eligibility, and a main visit approximately 1 week later, at which the measures of substance use were administered.

Setting: Dual-diagnosis program of a university-affiliated community mental health center.

Study design: Cross-sectional.

Overall risk of study bias: **High**

- **Selection bias:** *High Risk:* This study examined the concordance among self- and collateral reports of substance use, and urine toxicology screen results. Subjects who chose to be part of the study and allow collateral interviews may be more likely to discuss their substance use accurately, which may make them a nonrepresentative sample.
- **Performance bias:** *High Risk:* This study used a nonblinded cross-sectional design. Participants knew they were being interviewed and raters knew subjects' clinical characteristics, both of which may have affected the results.
- **Attrition bias:** *Unknown:* There were two study visits, one for a diagnostic interview and determination of eligibility, and the other for the baseline interview to collect substance use information. The authors noted that if a subject had a positive breath test for alcohol, the visit was rescheduled. No information is provided on rates of attrition between the two study visits.
- **Detection bias:** *High Risk:* Subjects and collateral sources may under- or overreport substance use. The authors noted the possibility that subject reports may have been influenced by the knowledge that collateral report and urine toxicology screening would be used for corroboration. Also, while the study measures had acceptable reliability and validity, reports of drug use were based on recall from memory.
- **Reporting bias:** *Low Risk:* There was no evidence of selective outcome reporting.
- **Sponsor-related bias:** *Low Risk:* This study was sponsored by National Institute on Alcohol Abuse and Alcoholism Grant R01 AA12805 to Clara M. Bradizza. There was no evidence that the sponsors or authors introduced bias into the results of the study.

Applicability: This study covers use of alcohol and other substances, but the setting was a specialized dual diagnosis program, and the subjects would be expected to have extremely high rates of substance use disorders, limiting the applicability of the study findings to other settings. The main goal of the study was to determine the agreement between different methods of substance use assessment, which makes its finding less applicable to the question of whether such assessment improves identification and diagnosis.

Grading of Supporting Body of Research Evidence

Risk of bias: **High Risk:** The body of evidence is made up of only observational studies, of varying quality.

Consistency: **Consistent:** The studies report that standardized questionnaires and collateral information are helpful in identifying risky drinking, alcohol use disorders, and substance use.

Directness: **Direct:** In these studies, use of enhanced detection methods (questionnaires or collateral sources) improved detection and diagnosis of alcohol disorders.

Precision: **Not applicable.**

Dose-response relationship: **Not applicable.**

Magnitude of effect: **Strong:** Using various enhancements to the standard clinical interview, whether a questionnaire or contacting a collateral source of information, appears to improve diagnosis, compared with clinical interviews or routine care.

Confounding factors (including likely direction of effect):   Patients who are willing to participate in studies about alcoholism and substance use may not be representative of all patients, because they may, on average, have lower amounts of substance use than those who do not wish to participate. Also, when filling out questionnaires, patients may not accurately represent their own alcohol or substance use. The expected effects of these issues is that the rates of drinking found in the studies are likely to be an underestimate of the amount of alcohol use disorders in the general public or among patients who present with psychiatric complaints.

Publication bias: **Not able to be assessed.**

Applicability: The body of evidence only addresses use of alcohol and some substances; it does not address misuse of over-the-counter and prescription medications. In addition, the settings in which the studies were conducted did not include the full scope of psychiatric settings. Two of the studies identified "at risk drinking" rather than a diagnosis of an alcohol use disorder per se. In one study, the questioning about alcohol use was not done in the context of an initial psychiatric interview, which limits the applicability of this study to the clinical question.

Overall strength of research evidence: **Low.**

Differences of Opinion in Rating the Strength of Recommendations

None.

Expert Opinion Data: Results

To what extent do you agree that the identification and diagnosis of substance use disorders is improved when the initial psychiatric evaluation of any patient typically (i.e., almost always) includes assessment of the following?

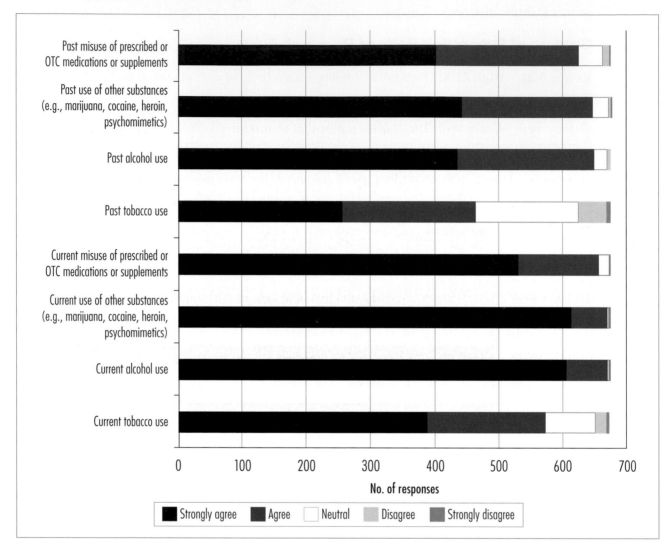

Percentage of experts who "strongly agreed" or "agreed" that the identification and diagnosis of substance use disorders is improved when the initial psychiatric evaluation of any patient typically (i.e., almost always) includes assessment of the following:

Past misuse of prescribed or over-the-counter (OTC) medications or supplements	92.6%
Past use of other substances (e.g., marijuana, cocaine, heroin, psychomimetics)	95.9%
Past alcohol use	96.2%
Past tobacco use	68.8%
Current misuse of prescribed or OTC medications or supplements	97.2%
Current use of other substances (e.g., marijuana, cocaine, heroin, psychomimetics)	99.7%
Current alcohol use	99.4%
Current tobacco use	85.6%

Do you typically (i.e., almost always) assess for the presence or absence of these items during initial evaluations of your patients?

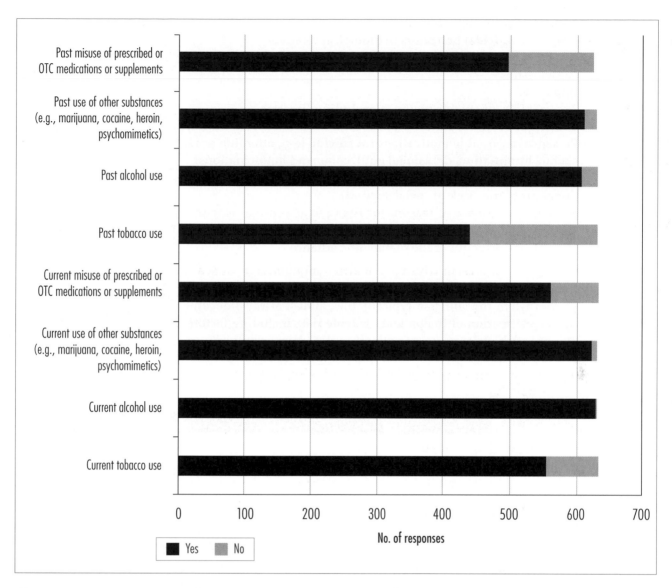

GUIDELINE III. Assessment of Suicide Risk

Clinical Questions

Development of this guideline was premised on the following clinical questions:

For patients who present with a psychiatric symptom, sign, or syndrome in any setting, is identification of risk for suicide improved when the initial psychiatric evaluation typically (i.e., almost always) includes assessment of the following?

- **Current suicidal ideas, including active or passive thoughts of suicide or death**
- **Current suicide plans**
- **Current suicide intent**
- **Intended course of action if current symptoms worsen**
- **Prior suicidal ideas or suicide plans**
- **Prior suicide attempts**

- Prior aborted or interrupted suicide attempts (in which an attempt was stopped by the individual or by someone else)
- Prior intentional self-injury without suicide intent
- History of psychiatric hospitalization
- History of suicidal behaviors in biological relatives
- Anxiety symptoms, including panic attacks
- Hopelessness
- Impulsivity
- Accessibility of suicide methods, including firearms
- Current or recent dependence, abuse, or increased use of alcohol or other substances
- Presence of possible motivations for suicide (e.g., attention or reaction from others, revenge, shame, humiliation, delusional guilt, command hallucinations)
- Presence or absence of psychosocial stressors (e.g., financial, housing, legal or school/occupational problems; lack of social support)
- Presence or absence of reasons for living (e.g., sense of responsibility to children or others, religious beliefs)
- Quality and strength of the therapeutic alliance

For patients who present with a psychiatric symptom, sign, or syndrome in any setting, is an individual clinician's decision making about a patient's psychiatric diagnosis and treatment plan improved when the clinician typically (i.e., almost always) documents in the patient's medical record an estimation of the patient's suicide risk, including factors influencing risk? Is coordination of psychiatric treatment with other clinicians improved?

Review of Supporting Research Evidence

Overview of Studies

Few studies have systematically assessed the benefits of a suicide risk assessment in reducing rates of suicide or suicide attempts.

A study by Pokorny (1983) examined the ability of multiple potential risk factors to predict later suicide or suicide attempts in 4,800 individuals who had been psychiatrically admitted to a Veterans Administration (VA) hospital in the United States and were followed for 4–6 years. Although some factors seemed to correlate with an increase in suicide risk, the ability of these risk factors (considered singly or together) to predict suicide or suicide attempts in particular individuals was low. This low positive predictive ability resulted in high numbers of false positives and false negatives, related in part to low sensitivity and specificity of the risk factors and in part to the relatively low population rates of suicide and suicide attempts. A reanalysis of these same data by Pokorny (1993), using logistic regression, confirmed that the positive predictive value of the identified risk factors was low.

Study	Subjects/Method	N	Design/ Duration	Outcomes
Pokorny 1983	Patients consecutively admitted to a VA hospital were part of the study. These patients underwent a series of risk assessment batteries at admission and then were followed for 4–6 years.	4,800	Prospective cohort study; patients followed for 4–6 years after the incident admission.	Despite using assessment instruments that had previously been reported to be predictive of suicide, the authors concluded that because of the low sensitivity and specificity of the instruments, and the low base rate of suicide itself, predicting which persons would later commit suicide would not be feasible.

No studies have addressed the benefits of documenting suicide risk in the medical record.

Grading of Quality of Individual Studies

Citation: Pokorny AD: Prediction of suicide in psychiatric patients: report of a Prospective Study. *Archives of General Psychiatry* 40(3):249–257, 1983

Population: 4,800 patients consecutively admitted to a VA hospital in Houston, Texas.

Intervention: Risk assessment battery was administered at the time of index admission.

Comparators: Not applicable.

Outcomes: Prediction of suicide or attempted suicide in particular individuals during a 4- to 6-year follow-up period was not feasible.

Timing: Administration of risk assessment battery at index admission, with follow-up for 4–6 years.

Setting: VA hospital, inpatient psychiatric service.

Study design: Prospective cohort study.

Study sponsorship: National Institute of Mental Health and VA research funds.

Overall risk of study bias: **Low**

- **Selection bias:** *Low Risk:* All patients were included in the sample and followed longitudinally.
- **Performance bias:** *Low Risk:* Given the longitudinal nature of the study, there is no reason to postulate a systematic difference in the care given to participants, and the initial interviewers were unaware of the subjects' ultimate outcome.
- **Attrition bias:** *Low Risk:* All 4,800 patients continued to be followed throughout the study.
- **Detection bias:** *Low Risk:* There was no attrition, and multiple approaches were used to determine whether patients had died during the study period (including by suicide) and/or had made a suicide attempt.
- **Reporting bias:** *Low Risk:* Initial assessments were done without knowledge of outcome, and the outcomes were binary in nature.
- **Sponsor-related bias:** *Low Risk:* The study had a noncommercial funding source, and there were no obvious sources of other investigator bias.

Applicability: The study population consists of only psychiatric inpatients. There are some limits on generalizability of the findings given the differences between VA hospital populations and general psychiatric inpatient unit populations.

Grading of Supporting Body of Research Evidence

Risk of bias: **High Risk:** The body of evidence consists of only one observational study with a sample size that was too small to overcome issues with the low base rate of suicide.

Consistency: Consistency cannot be determined because there is only one study.

Directness: **Direct:** The study examined the effect of a risk assessment battery on prediction of suicide in psychiatric patients.

Precision: **Imprecise:** Because of the low base rate of suicide and small sample size, the estimate of effect does not suggest a clinically useful conclusion.

Dose-response relationship: **Not applicable.**

Magnitude of effect: **Weak.**

Confounding factors (including likely direction of effect): **Absent.**

Publication bias: **Not able to be assessed.**

Applicability: The study involved VA hospital inpatients, who were mostly male.

Overall strength of research evidence: **Low.**

Differences of Opinion in Rating the Strength of Recommendations

One member of the work group was uncertain about the value of assessing two risk factors: hopelessness and impulsivity. In patients who report current suicidal ideas, one member of the work group was uncertain about the value of assessing the patient's reasons for living. These are considered to be minor differences of opinion.

Expert Opinion Data: Results

To what extent do you agree that identification of patients at risk for suicide is improved when the initial psychiatric evaluation of any patient typically (i.e., almost always) includes assessment of the following?

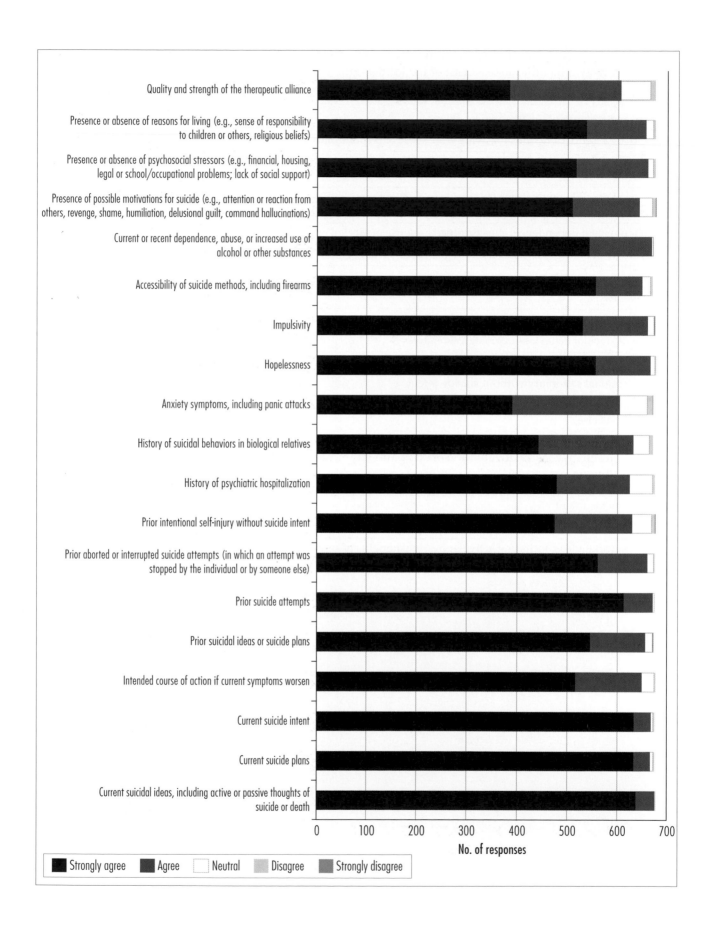

Percentage of experts who "strongly agreed" or "agreed" that identification of patients at risk for suicide is improved when the initial psychiatric evaluation of any patient typically (i.e., almost always) includes assessment of the following:

Quality and strength of the therapeutic alliance	89.9%
Presence or absence of reasons for living (e.g., sense of responsibility to children or others, religious beliefs)	97.3%
Presence or absence of psychosocial stressors (e.g., financial, housing, legal or school/occupational problems; lack of social support)	98.1%
Presence of possible motivations for suicide (e.g., attention or reaction from others, revenge, shame, humiliation, delusional guilt, command hallucinations)	95.3%
Current or recent dependence, abuse, or increased use of alcohol or other substances	99.6%
Accessibility of suicide methods, including firearms	96.7%
Impulsivity	97.8%
Hopelessness	98.7%
Anxiety symptoms, including panic attacks	89.6%
History of suicidal behaviors in biological relatives	94.0%
History of psychiatric hospitalization	92.5%
Prior intentional self-injury without suicide intent	93.2%
Prior aborted or interrupted suicide attempts (in which an attempt was stopped by the individual or by someone else)	97.8%
Prior suicide attempts	99.7%
Prior suicidal ideas or suicide plans	97.6%
Intended course of action if current symptoms worsen	96.0%
Current suicide intent	99.1%
Current suicide plans	99.1%
Current suicidal ideas, including active or passive thoughts of suicide or death	99.7%

Do you typically (i.e., almost always) assess these items during initial evaluations of your patients?

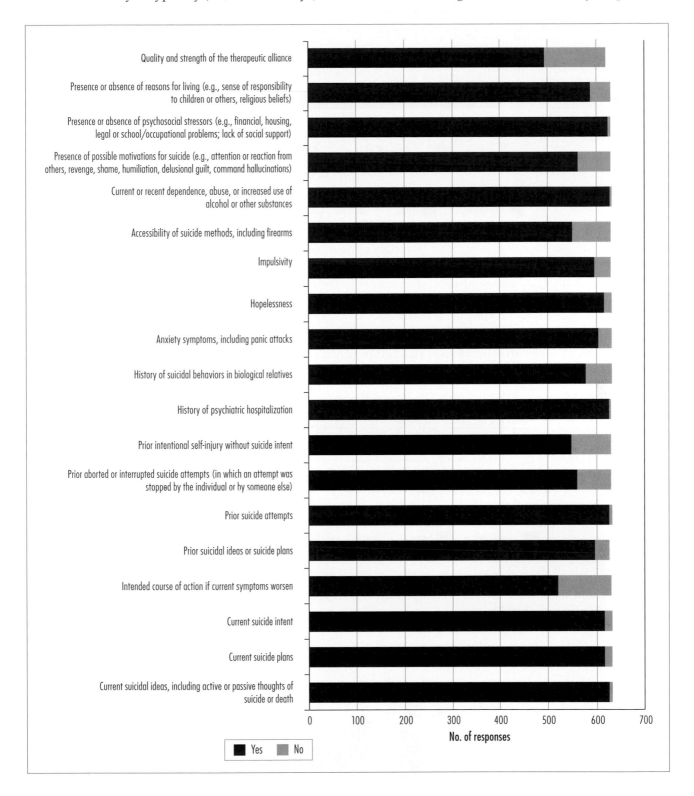

To what extent do you agree that an individual clinician's decision making about a patient's psychiatric diagnosis and treatment plan is improved when the clinician typically (i.e., almost always) documents in the patient's medical record an estimation of suicide risk, including factors influencing risk?

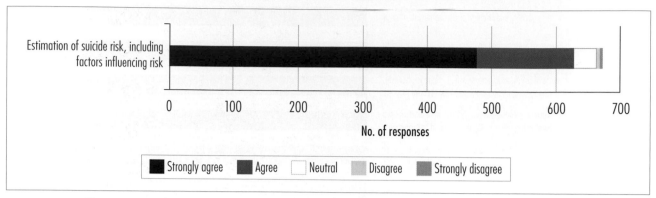

Percentage of experts who "strongly agreed" or "agreed" that an individual clinician's decision making about a patient's psychiatric diagnosis and treatment plan is improved when the clinician typically (i.e., almost always) documents in the patient's medical record an estimation of suicide risk, including factors influencing risk: 93.2%.

To what extent do you agree that coordination of psychiatric treatment with other clinicians is improved when an estimation of risk is typically (i.e., almost always) documented?

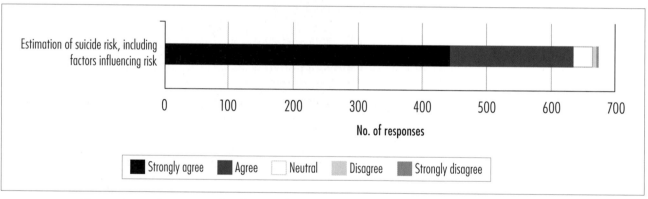

Percentage of experts who "strongly agreed" or "agreed" that coordination of psychiatric treatment with other clinicians is improved when an estimation of risk is typically (i.e., almost always) documented: 94.5%.

Do you typically (i.e., almost always) document an estimation of risk in the medical record of your patients?

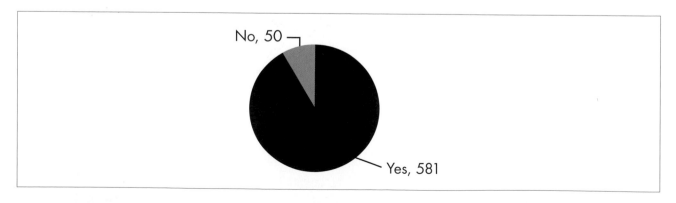

GUIDELINE IV. Assessment of Risk for Aggressive Behaviors

Clinical Questions

Development of this guideline was premised on the following clinical questions:

For patients who present with a psychiatric symptom, sign, or syndrome in any setting, is identification of risk for aggressive behaviors improved when the initial psychiatric evaluation typically (i.e., almost always) includes assessment of the following?

- Current aggressive ideas, including thoughts of physical or sexual aggression or homicide
- Prior homicidal or aggressive behaviors, including domestic or workplace violence or other physically or sexually aggressive threats or acts
- Prior homicidal or aggressive ideas
- History of psychiatric emergency visits or psychiatric hospitalization
- Legal or disciplinary consequences of aggressive behaviors, including school expulsion, arrests, or orders of protection
- Current or recent dependence, abuse, or increased use of alcohol or other substances
- Impulsivity, including anger management issues
- Access to firearms
- Psychosocial stressors (e.g., financial situation, housing/homelessness, lack of social support)
- Family history of abuse or violence
- Exposure to violence or aggressive behavior, including combat exposure
- Neurological disorder (e.g., traumatic brain injury, seizure)

For patients who present with a psychiatric symptom, sign, or syndrome in any setting, is an individual clinician's decision making about a patient's psychiatric diagnosis and treatment plan improved when the clinician typically (i.e., almost always) documents in the patient's medical record an estimation of risk of aggressive behavior (including homicide), including factors influencing risk? Is coordination of psychiatric treatment with other clinicians improved?

Review of Supporting Research Evidence

Overview of Studies

Study	Subjects/Method	N	Design/ Duration	Outcomes
Abderhalden et al. 2008	Fourteen acute psychiatric units in Switzerland were randomly assigned to provide a structured nursing risk assessment for all new admissions (four units) vs. wait-list control (five units). Five other units elected to provide the assessment without entering randomization. The assessment produces a risk score from 0 to 12.	2,364	Randomized controlled trial; June 2002 through April 2004.	In the units performing the risk assessments, there was a 41% reduction in severe aggressive incidents and a 27% decline in the use of coercive measures. The severity of incidents did not decrease. The authors concluded that structured risk assessment during the first days of treatment may contribute to reduced violence and coercion in acute psychiatric wards.
Van de Sande et al. 2011	Four acute psychiatric units in a single hospital in the Netherlands were randomly assigned to use either a structured risk assessment on all admitted patients (two units) or clinical judgment of risk (two units).	597	Randomized controlled trial; 10 weeks pre-randomization lead-in period and 30-week study period; dates unreported.	In the units performing structured risk assessments, there was a 68% decrease in the number of aggressive incidents. Hours spent in seclusion also declined in the intervention group (by 45%). The authors concluded that structured risk assessment may help reduce aggressive incidents and use of restraint and seclusion in acute psychiatric wards.

Grading of Quality of Individual Studies

Citation: Abderhalden C, Needham I, Dassen T, et al.: Structured risk assessment and violence in acute psychiatric wards: randomised controlled trial. *British Journal of Psychiatry* 193(1):44–50, 2008

Population: Patients in psychiatric units in Switzerland. There were 324 psychiatric units in the area that were screened on eligibility criteria (i.e., majority of patients have an acute psychiatric disorder, patients are admitted directly onto the unit, patients usually stay less than 3 months, patients are 18–65 years old, and the unit admits all potential patients and is not specialized for the treatment of specific disorders). Out of the 324 units, 86 met these criteria and were invited to participate. Sixty-two units declined participation. Nine units were randomized to the intervention or wait-list control; five units elected to use the intervention without undergoing randomization. A total of 2,364 patients were admitted across the 14 units (46.6% female, mean age=39.5 years, SD=14.2, range=14–95). Of these patients, 56% were admitted voluntarily, a rate of voluntary admission that is typical for the area. Approximately 24% of patients had disorders due to psychoactive substance use; 31% had schizophrenia, schizotypal, or delusional disorders; and 16% had mood disorders.

Intervention: All patients in the intervention units received a nurse-administered structured short-term risk assessment within 3 days of admission to the unit. The assessment was the previously validated extended Swiss version of the Broset Violence Checklist (BVC-CH). The checklist rates six patient behaviors (confusion, irritability, boisterousness, verbal threats, physical threats, and attacks on objects) and includes an overall subjective assessment of the risk of imminent violence using a slide-rule visual analogue scale. The ratings are combined to produce a score between 0 (very low risk) and 12 (high risk).

Comparators: Wait-list control and preference group. Data from the 3-month baseline period were compared with those from the 3-month intervention period for each group.

Outcomes: Incidence rates of aggressive behaviors decreased in the intervention units but were unchanged in control units. The overall incidence rate of severe aggressive events was 1.09 (95% confidence interval [CI] 0.96–1.24) per 100 hospitalization days during the 3-month baseline period as compared with 0.75 (95% CI 0.65–0.87) during the 3-month intervention period. For the use of coercive measures (e.g., emergency medication treatment, seclusion, restraint), the overall incidence rate was 1.57 (95% CI 1.41–1.75) per 100 hospitalization days during the baseline and 1.20 (95% CI 1.07–1.35) during the intervention period. Decline in severe aggressive events in the intervention units (adjusted risk ratio=0.59, 95% CI 0.41–0.83) was significantly larger ($P<0.001$) than the decline in the control units (RR=0.85, 95% CI 0.63–1.13). Rates declined more in intervention units than in control units for both secondary outcomes: attacks (41% vs. 7%; $P<0.001$) and use of coercive measures (27% vs. increase of 10%; $P<0.001$). Effects were larger in the preference units than in the randomized units (attacks: 64% decline, coercive measures: 60% decline).

Timing: The first unit was enrolled in June 2002, and the last unit completed the study in April 2004. Baseline data were collected in all units over a 3-month period, followed by a 3-month intervention period.

Setting: Psychiatric inpatient units in the German-speaking area of Switzerland.

Study design: Randomized controlled trial (psychiatric units served as the unit of randomization).

Overall risk of study bias: **Moderate**

- **Selection bias:** *High Risk:* The investigators conducted a survey of all units in the area prior to the study in order to control for recruitment bias. Survey questions inquired about unit size, staffing, facilities for managing aggression and violence, leaders' ratings of the severity of the problem, and resources for aggression management. The leaders of intervention units rated aggression as a greater problem than leaders of other units. The baseline rates of aggression were higher in the intervention units than in the control units. The preference units had significantly fewer patients with diagnoses of schizophrenia, schizotypal, or delusional disorders than the randomized units. The distribution of diagnoses across the intervention and control arms was comparable. No other differences reported.
- **Performance bias:** *Moderate Risk:* Neither raters nor patients were blinded to intervention condition. There is no evidence of systematic differences in treatment of the study groups.
- **Attrition bias:** *Moderate Risk:* Sixty-two psychiatric units declined participation. It is possible that these units differed systematically from those that agreed to participate.
- **Detection bias:** *Low Risk:* All patients were included, and all aggressive incidents and rates of use of coercive measures were recorded. Two of the investigators regularly visited the units on randomly selected dates to review study data and ensure accurate recording. Underreporting of less severe incidents appeared to be more common as the study progressed, but no underreporting of severe incidents was noted.
- **Reporting bias:** *Low Risk:* There is no evidence of selective outcome reporting.

- **Sponsor-related bias:** *Low Risk:* The study was funded by a grant from the Swiss National Science Foundation. There is no evidence of sponsor-related bias.

Applicability: This study was conducted in acute inpatient psychiatric units in Switzerland, thus limiting generalizability of its findings to other treatment settings and to patients in the United States.

Citation: van de Sande R, Nijman HL, Noorthoorn EO, et al.: Aggression and seclusion on acute psychiatric wards: effect of short-term risk assessment. *British Journal of Psychiatry* **199(6):473–478, 2011**

Population: Patients in psychiatric units in the Netherlands. Four acute wards of a hospital in Rotterdam were randomized to conduct structured risk assessments on all admissions (2 units) or to use standard clinical judgments of risk (2 units). Of the 597 patients admitted during the trial, 62% were admitted involuntarily. Diagnostically, 58% of patients had a psychotic disorder and 18% had a personality disorder. The average age was 38.8 years, and 60% of the patients were male.

Intervention: All patients in the intervention units received a nurse-administered structured short-term risk assessments (the Broset Violence Checklist and the Kennedy Axis V–Short Version) on a daily basis, with the full version of the Kennedy Axis V scale, the Brief Psychiatric Rating Scale (BPRS), Dangerousness Scale, and Social Dysfunction and Aggression Scale administered on a weekly basis the results and discussed during meetings of the staff. Ratings were used to recognize early patterns of symptom evolution and behavioral escalation.

Comparators: Clinical judgment only. Data from the 10-week baseline period were compared with those from the 30-week intervention period for each group.

Outcomes: In the intervention period, as compared with the baseline, there was a significant decrease in the numbers of aggressive incidents (relative risk reduction [RRR] compared with controls of -68%, $P<0.001$), number of patients engaging in aggression (RRR$=-50\%$, $P<0.05$), and time spent in seclusion (RRR$=-45\%$, $P<0.05$). The weekly rate of aggressive incidents also decreased on the intervention unit, with an average of 4.9 incidents per week during the baseline period and an average of 1.7 incidents per week during the intervention period. In contrast, the number of aggressive incidents on the control unit did not change significantly during the baseline and intervention periods (3.5 incidents per week and 3.9 incidents per week, respectively). The number of seclusion episodes and the number of patients receiving seclusion did not differ between the intervention and control groups.

Timing: Study dates were not reported. Baseline data were collected in all units over a 10-week period, followed by a 30-week intervention period.

Setting: Psychiatric inpatient units in Rotterdam, The Netherlands.

Study design: Randomized controlled trial (psychiatric units served as the unit of randomization).

Overall risk of study bias: **Moderate**

- **Selection bias:** *High Risk:* As compared with the two units that were using standard clinical judgments of risk, the two units that were randomly assigned to implement structured risk assessments had a greater proportion of patients who had been admitted involuntarily and a greater proportion of patients with psychosis or a personality disorder. These differences were noted during the baseline period as well as during the time of the intervention.

- **Performance bias:** *Moderate Risk:* Neither raters nor patients were blinded to intervention condition. There is no evidence of systematic differences in treatment of the study groups.
- **Attrition bias:** *Low Risk:* All units continued to participate throughout the study, and patients on each unit remained in the study throughout their hospital stay.
- **Detection bias:** *Low Risk:* All patients were included, and all aggressive incidents and episodes of seclusion were recorded. Clinical nurse specialists visited all units on a daily basis to ensure that events were recorded consistently.
- **Reporting bias:** *Low Risk:* There is no evidence of selective outcome reporting.
- **Sponsor-related bias:** *Low Risk:* The study was funded by a grant from the Dutch Ministry of Health. There is no evidence of sponsor-related bias.

Applicability: This study was conducted in acute inpatient psychiatric units in the Netherlands, thus limiting generalizability of the findings to other treatment settings and to patients in the United States.

Grading of Supporting Body of Research Evidence

Risk of bias: **High Risk:** The body of evidence consists of two nonblinded studies, with a total of 13 psychiatric units randomly assigned to intervention or control.

Consistency: **Consistent:** Both studies showed reductions in incidents of aggressive behavior and in use of seclusion and/or restraint.

Directness: **Indirect:** Although the studies did measure specific aggressive behaviors as one outcome, the specific risk assessment elements used in the study were not the same as those outlined in the clinical question.

Precision: **Precise:** Confidence intervals reported in the studies were fairly narrow.

Dose-response relationship: **Not applicable.**

Magnitude of effect: **Weak:** Although there were significant declines in aggressive events, some or all of this change could have resulted from other unmeasured changes (e.g., staff behavior) that would have also affected rates of aggressive events.

Confounding factors that would decrease the magnitude of the effect: **Absent.**

Publication bias: **Not able to be assessed.**

Applicability: The two study samples comprised psychiatric inpatients at European hospitals, limiting the applicability of the findings to other settings. Also, the assessment did not address all assessment items in the clinical question.

Overall strength of research evidence: **Low.**

Differences of Opinion in Rating the Strength of Recommendations

One work group member was uncertain about the benefits of assessing for neurological disorder. On all other aspects of these recommendations, work group opinion was unanimous.

Expert Opinion Data: Results

To what extent do you agree that identification of patients at risk for aggressive behaviors is improved when the initial psychiatric evaluation of any patient typically (i.e., almost always) includes assessment of the following?

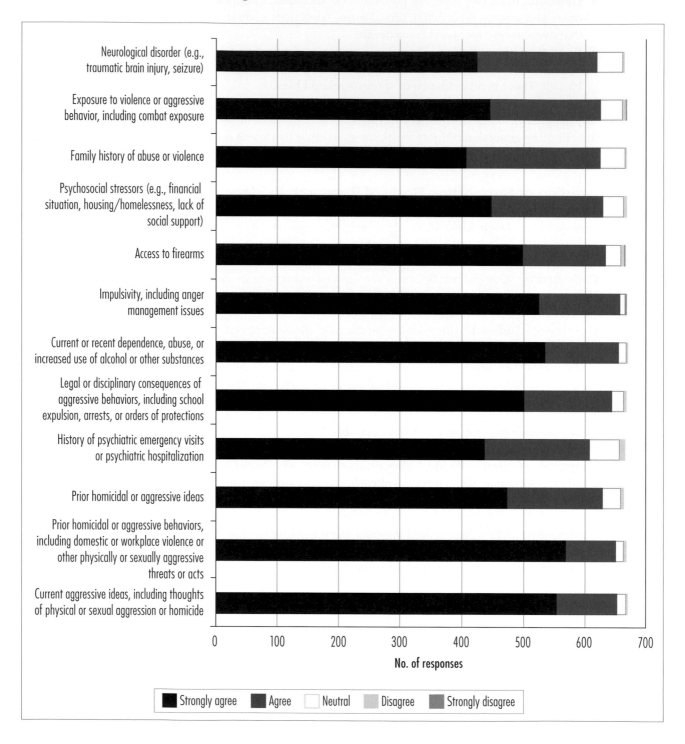

Percentage of experts who "strongly agreed" or "agreed" that identification of patients at risk for aggressive behaviors is improved when the initial psychiatric evaluation of any patient typically (i.e., almost always) includes assessment of the following:

Neurological disorder (e.g., traumatic brain injury, seizure)	93.5%
Exposure to violence or aggressive behavior, including combat exposure	93.7%
Family history of abuse or violence	93.7%
Psychosocial stressors (e.g., financial situation, housing/homelessness, lack of social support)	94.3%
Access to firearms	95.3%
Impulsivity, including anger management issues	98.4%
Current or recent dependence, abuse, or increased use of alcohol or other substances	98.1%
Legal or disciplinary consequences of aggressive behaviors, including school expulsion, arrests, or orders of protection	96.7%
History of psychiatric emergency visits or psychiatric hospitalization	91.4%
Prior homicidal or aggressive ideas	94.7%
Prior homicidal or aggressive behaviors, including domestic or workplace violence or other physically or sexually aggressive threats or acts	97.9%
Current aggressive ideas, including thoughts of physical or sexual aggression or homicide	97.8%

Do you typically (i.e., almost always) assess these items during initial evaluations of your patients?

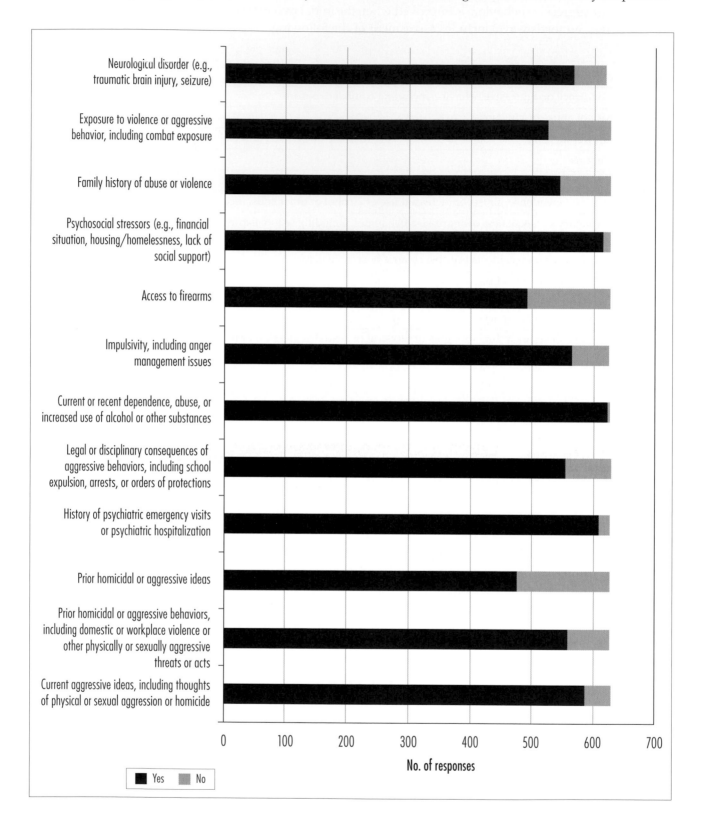

APA Practice Guidelines

To what extent do you agree that an individual clinician's decision making about a patient's psychiatric diagnosis and treatment plan is improved when the clinician typically (i.e., almost always) documents in the patient's medical record an estimation of risk of aggressive behavior, including factors influencing risk?

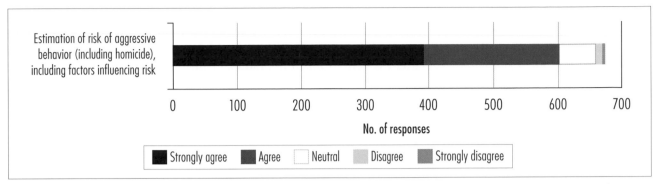

Percentage of experts who "strongly agreed" or "agreed" that an individual clinician's decision making about a patient's psychiatric diagnosis and treatment plan is improved when the clinician typically (i.e., almost always) documents in the patient's medical record an estimation of risk of aggressive behavior, including factors influencing risk: 89.3%.

To what extent do you agree that coordination of psychiatric treatment with other clinicians is improved when an estimation of risk of aggressive behavior, including factors influencing risk, is typically (i.e., almost always) documented?

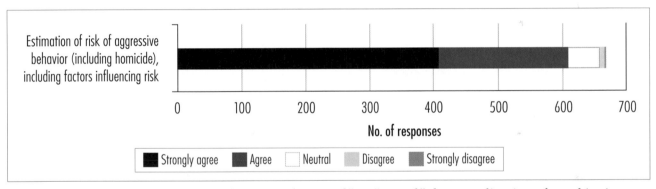

Percentage of experts who "strongly agreed" or "agreed" that coordination of psychiatric treatment with other clinicians is improved when an estimation of risk of aggressive behavior, including factors influencing risk, is typically (i.e., almost always) documented: 91.3%.

Do you typically (i.e., almost always) document an estimation of risk of aggressive behavior, including factors influencing risk, in the medical record of your patients?

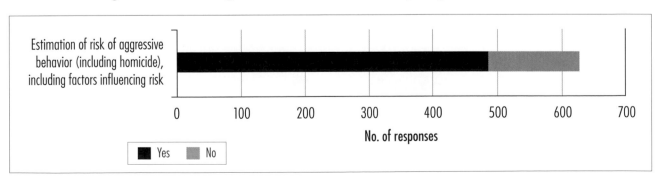

GUIDELINE V. Assessment of Cultural Factors

Clinical Questions

Development of this guideline was premised on the following clinical questions:

For patients who present with a psychiatric symptom, sign, or syndrome in any setting, is formulation of an appropriate treatment plan improved when the initial psychiatric evaluation typically (i.e., almost always) includes assessment of his or her language needs (i.e., basic language ability and need for an interpreter)?

For patients who present with a psychiatric symptom, sign, or syndrome in any setting, are the therapeutic alliance, accuracy of diagnosis, and formulation of an appropriate treatment plan improved when the initial psychiatric evaluation typically (i.e., almost always) includes assessment of his or her personal/cultural beliefs?

For patients who present with a psychiatric symptom, sign, or syndrome in any setting, are the therapeutic alliance, accuracy of diagnosis, and formulation of an appropriate treatment plan improved when the initial psychiatric evaluation typically (i.e., almost always) includes assessment of his or her cultural explanations of psychiatric illness?

For patients who present with a psychiatric symptom, sign, or syndrome in any setting, are the therapeutic alliance, accuracy of diagnosis, and formulation of an appropriate treatment plan improved when the initial psychiatric evaluation typically (i.e., almost always) includes assessment of cultural factors related to his or her social environment (e.g., family network, workplace, religious group, community, or other psychosocial support network)?

Review of Supporting Research Evidence

Overview of Studies

There is no supporting research evidence that specifically addresses the above clinical questions.

Grading of Quality of Individual Studies

Not applicable.

Grading of Supporting Body of Research Evidence

Not applicable.

Differences of Opinion in Rating the Strength of Recommendations

One member of the work group was uncertain that potential benefits of assessing cultural factors related to the patient's social environment clearly outweigh harms. This difference of opinion is considered minor.

Expert Opinion Data: Results

To what extent do you agree that formulation of an appropriate treatment plan is improved when the initial psychiatric evaluation of any patient typically (i.e., almost always) includes assessment of the patient's language needs (i.e., basic language ability and need for an interpreter)?

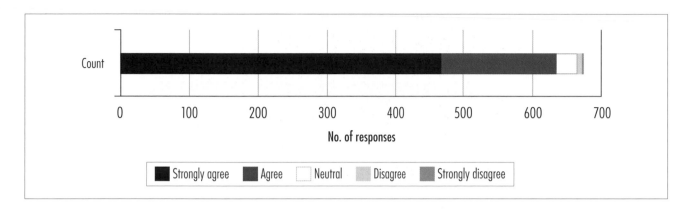

Percentage of experts who "strongly agreed" or "agreed" that formulation of an appropriate treatment plan is improved when the initial psychiatric evaluation of any patient typically (i.e., almost always) includes assessment of the patient's language needs: 94.2%.

Do you typically (i.e., almost always) assess your patients' language needs during initial psychiatric evaluations?

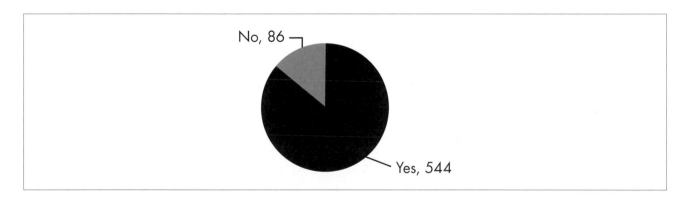

To what extent do you agree that the following are improved when the initial psychiatric evaluation of any patient typically (i.e., almost always) includes assessment of his or her personal/cultural beliefs?[5]

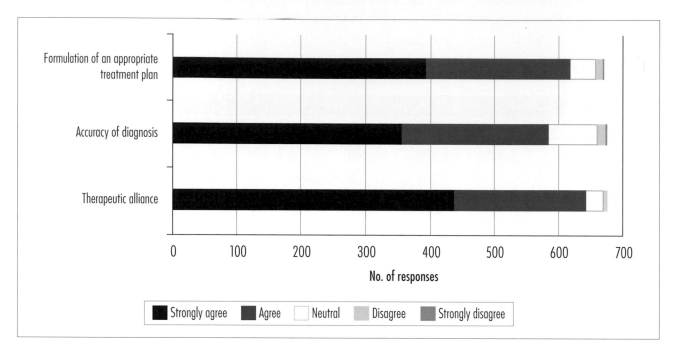

Percentage of experts who "strongly agreed" or "agreed" that the following are improved when the initial psychiatric evaluation of any patient typically (i.e., almost always) includes assessment of his or her personal/cultural beliefs:

Therapeutic alliance	95.3%
Accuracy of diagnosis	86.6%
Formulation of an appropriate treatment plan	92.7%

Do you typically (i.e., almost always) assess your patients' personal/cultural beliefs during initial psychiatric evaluations?

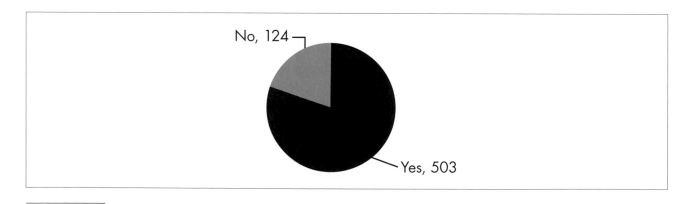

---

[5] Personal/cultural beliefs are defined as beliefs related to the patient's personal/cultural characteristics and identity, including but not limited to beliefs about age, ethnicity, gender, race, religion, and sexuality.

To what extent do you agree that the following are improved when the initial psychiatric evaluation of any patient typically (i.e., almost always) includes assessment of his or her cultural explanations of psychiatric illness?

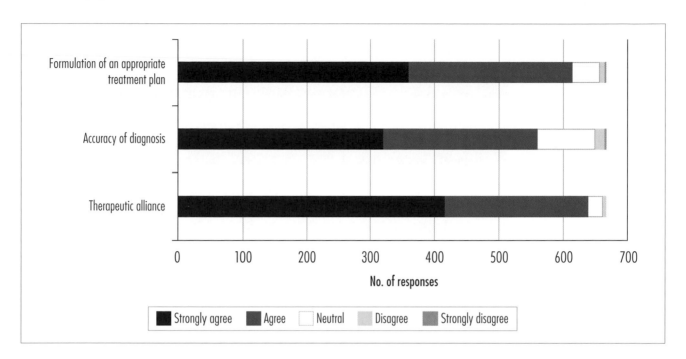

Percentage of experts who "strongly agreed" or "agreed" that the following are improved when the initial psychiatric evaluation of any patient typically (i.e., almost always) includes assessment of his or her cultural explanations of psychiatric illness:

Formulation of an appropriate treatment plan	92.7%
Accuracy of diagnosis	84.1%
Therapeutic alliance	96.0%

Do you typically (i.e., almost always) assess your patients' cultural explanations of their psychiatric illness during initial psychiatric evaluations?

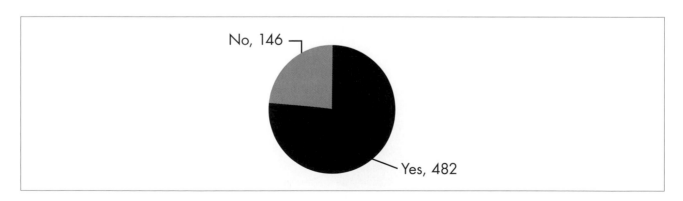

To what extent do you agree that the following are improved when the initial psychiatric evaluation of any patient typically (i.e., almost always) includes assessment of cultural factors related to his or her social environment (e.g., family network, religious group, community, or other social support network)?

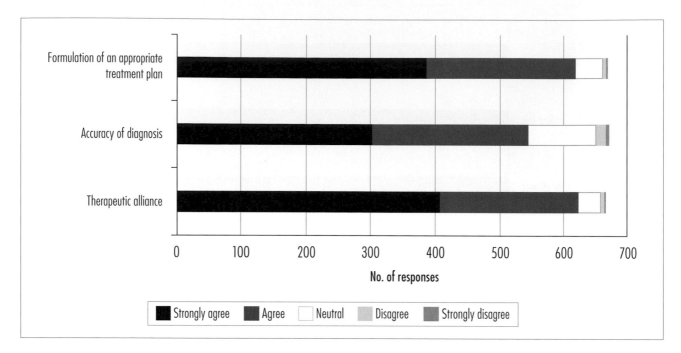

Percentage of experts who "strongly agreed" or "agreed" that the following are improved when the initial psychiatric evaluation of any patient typically (i.e., almost always) includes assessment of cultural factors related to his or her social environment:

Formulation of an appropriate treatment plan	92.7%
Accuracy of diagnosis	81.5%
Therapeutic alliance	93.7%

Do you typically (i.e., almost always) include in initial psychiatric evaluations assessment of cultural factors related to your patients' social environment?

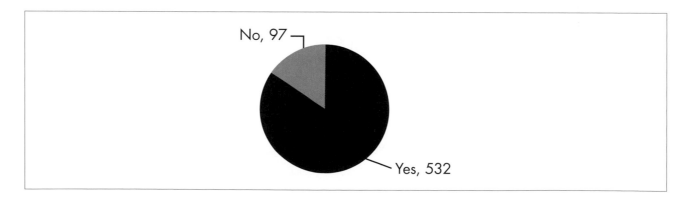

GUIDELINE VI. Assessment of Medical Health

Clinical Questions

Development of this guideline was premised on the following clinical questions:

For patients who present with a psychiatric symptom, sign, or syndrome in any setting, should an initial psychiatric evaluation typically (i.e., almost always) include assessment of whether or not the patient has an ongoing relationship with a primary care health professional?

For patients who present with a psychiatric symptom, sign, or syndrome in any setting, are diagnostic accuracy and treatment safety improved when the initial psychiatric evaluation typically (i.e., almost always) includes assessment of the following aspects of the patient's *current general medical status*? "Assessment" is defined here as a) performing a physical examination on the patient, b) directing another clinician (e.g., a resident) to perform the exam, or c) reviewing the results of a recent physical examination performed by another clinician.

a. General appearance and nutritional status
b. Height, weight, body mass index (BMI)
c. Vital signs
d. Skin, including any stigmata of trauma, self-injury, or drug use
e. Cardiopulmonary status
f. Involuntary movements or abnormalities of motor tone
g. Coordination and gait
h. Speech, including fluency and articulation
i. Cranial nerves, including sight and hearing
j. Reflexes and peripheral motor and sensory functions

For patients who present with a psychiatric symptom, sign, or syndrome in any setting, are diagnostic accuracy and treatment safety improved when the initial psychiatric evaluation typically (i.e., almost always) includes assessment of the following aspects of the patient's *general medical history*? Assessment may occur directly or by review of the results of a recent assessment by another clinician.

a. Physical trauma, including head injuries
b. Past or current general medical illnesses and related hospitalizations
c. Important past or current treatments or procedures, including complementary and alternative medical treatments
d. Allergies or drug sensitivities
e. Past or current endocrinological disease
f. Past or current infectious disease, including but not limited to sexually transmitted diseases, HIV, tuberculosis, and hepatitis C
g. Past or current neurological disorders or symptoms
h. Sexual and reproductive history
i. Past or current sleep disorders, including sleep apnea
j. Past or current symptoms or conditions associated with significant pain and discomfort

For patients who present with a psychiatric symptom, sign, or syndrome in any setting, are diagnostic accuracy and treatment safety improved when the initial psychiatric evaluation typically (i.e., almost always) includes review of all medications the patient is currently or recently taking and the side effects of these medications? "All medications" means both prescribed and nonprescribed medications, herbal and nutritional supplements, and vitamins.

For patients who present with a psychiatric symptom, sign, or syndrome in any setting, are diagnostic accuracy and treatment safety improved when the initial psychiatric evaluation typically (i.e., almost always) includes the following elements of a review of systems?

a. General/systemic
b. Skin
c. HEENT (head, ears, eyes, nose, throat)
d. Respiratory
e. Cardiovascular
f. Gastrointestinal
g. Genitourinary
h. Musculoskeletal
i. Neurological
j. Hematological
k. Endocrine

Review of Supporting Research Evidence

Overview of Studies

Few studies have examined the role of medical assessment in improving diagnostic accuracy or treatment safety within the context of an initial psychiatric evaluation (i.e., across a broad range of patient characteristics or settings). Available studies have typically examined the ability of a screening history, physical examination, or battery of tests on the identification of medical causes of psychiatric symptoms.

Study	Subjects/Method	N	Design/ Duration	Outcomes
Hall et al. 1981	100 state hospital psychiatric patients consecutively admitted to a research ward were screened for physical illness prior to admission.	100	Observational study; duration not specified in the study.	46% of these patients had an unrecognized medical illness that either caused or exacerbated their psychiatric illness. 80% had physical illness requiring treatment, and 4% had precancerous conditions or illnesses. The authors suggested that a physical exam and a battery of medical screening tests be part of a routine workup for all hospitalized psychiatric patients.

Study	Subjects/Method	N	Design/Duration	Outcomes
Henneman et al. 1994	A medical history, physical examination, lab work, computed tomography (CT) scan, lumbar puncture (LP) if febrile, and a psychiatric evaluation were completed on 100 consecutive patients with new psychiatric symptoms, ages 16–65, who presented to an urban, county hospital. Exclusion criteria: obvious alcohol or drug intoxication, prior psychiatric diagnosis, patients with medical complaints who overdosed or attempted suicide.	100	Cohort study; 9-month period	Results were considered significant when they identified an etiology for the symptoms or resulted in medical admission. 63 of the 100 patients had an organic etiology for their psychiatric symptoms. The medical history was significant in 27, physical examination in 6, alcohol and drug screen in 28; complete blood count (CBC) in 5, basic metabolic panel (SMA-7) in 10, creatine phosphokinase (CPK) in 6, LP in 3, and CT in 8. The authors concluded, "Most alert, adult patients with new psychiatric symptoms have an organic etiology." This particular battery of tests was recommended to obtain medical clearance.
Bartsch et al. 1990	175 patients from two community mental health centers in Colorado received physical exams and lab work.	175	Nonblinded observational study with a comparison control group; February–May 1985	20% had a previously undiagnosed physical health problem, 16% had conditions that could cause or exacerbate their mental disorder, and 46% had physical conditions or laboratory test results warranting further medical evaluation. The authors concluded that public mental health systems should ensure routine assessment of the physical health of psychiatric outpatients.

Grading of Quality of Individual Studies

Citation: Hall RC, Gardner ER, Popkin MK, et al.: Unrecognized physical illness prompting psychiatric admission: a prospective study. *American Journal of Psychiatry* **138(5):629–635, 1981**

Population: 100 consecutive involuntary patients who had been brought to an "urban psychiatric receiving unit" in Texas who "in all probability would have been committed to the state hospital" but were offered voluntary admission to a research unit for the study. Patients with known physical disorders were excluded, as were patients with "sociopathic personality disorders" and significant histories of drug or alcohol abuse.

Intervention: Patients received a physical examination by a general practitioner, tests of sight and hearing, computerized medical questionnaire, SMA-12, and an ECG. Within 24 hours of voluntary admission to the research unit, two additional detailed physical exams and a separate structured neurological exam were completed along with SMA-34 blood chemistry, EEG, urine drug screen, and routine urinalysis. Within 5 days of admission, a detailed life history questionnaire was completed and a battery of psychological tests was administered. Patients were referred to a university-based diagnostic group for complete workup if any diagnostic confusion existed.

Comparators: None.

Outcomes: Proportion of individuals who were found to have a previously unrecognized and undiagnosed medical illness that was felt to be specifically causing or exacerbating their psychiatric symptoms. Such an illness was detected in 46 patients (46%), of whom 28 were noted to have experienced "dramatic and rapid" clearing of their psychiatric symptoms when appropriate medical treatment was instituted.

Timing: Assessment occurred after patients' arrival at an urban psychiatric receiving unit and after their consent to voluntary admission to a research unit. Patients had been brought to the receiving unit on a mental health warrant.

Setting: Urban psychiatric receiving unit in Texas followed by voluntary admission to a research unit.

Study design: Observational study.

Study sponsorship: Not listed.

Overall risk of study bias: **Medium**

- **Selection bias:** *High Risk:* The patients selected were brought on a mental health warrant, and so they are likely more seriously mentally ill, with associated poorer medical health, than the general population—or even the general psychiatric population. Also, the study appears to indicate that patients were offered voluntary admission to a research unit, and it is unclear if patients may have had a legal incentive to do this, given the warrant they were brought in under. There is also a risk that the most severely ill patients were unable to provide informed consent and thus were not analyzed in the study. The authors noted that the patients would have been admitted to the state hospital if they had not been admitted to the research unit and may have had a different expectation of care or facilities.
- **Performance bias:** *Low Risk:* The assessments were performed consistently with the entire study population.
- **Attrition bias:** *Low Risk:* Patients were admitted and kept for the duration of the assessment. There is no mention of attrition in the study.
- **Detection bias:** *High Risk:* Determination of whether a test result is causally related to a patient's psychiatric presentation is a subjective clinical judgment and could be biased by investigators' hypotheses.
- **Reporting bias:** *Low Risk:* There is no evidence of systematic differences between reported and unreported findings. The authors listed disorders that were detected but did not seem to be related to the psychiatric symptoms in addition to those judged to be causing or exacerbating psychiatric symptoms, which reduces unseen bias.
- **Sponsor-related bias:** *Unclear,* as sponsorship is not specified.

Applicability: This study is limited by setting (urban psychiatric receiving unit) and patient population (involuntary patients). The age of the study may also limit its applicability in terms of changes in the healthcare delivery system, laboratory assessments, and the typical characteristics of individuals who present for an involuntary admission.

Citation: Henneman PL, Mendoza R, Lewis RJ: Prospective evaluation of emergency department medical clearance. *Annals of Emergency Medicine* **24(4):672–677, 1994**

Population: 100 consecutive patients (ages 16–65, 63 men and 37 women, with 40 Caucasian, 28 African American, and 30 Hispanic individuals) who presented with new psychiatric symptoms (hallucinations in 49%, agitation in 66%, disorientation in 60%) and who did not have obvious alcohol or drug intoxication, a prior psychiatric diagnosis, medical complaints, or a presentation with an overdose or attempted suicide.

Intervention: The following were carried out for each patient: a medical history; physical examination; alcohol level; urine screen for cocaine, amphetamine, and phencyclidine; CBC; SMA-7 (electrolytes, blood urea nitrogen, creatinine, glucose); calcium; CPK (if a urine dipstick was positive for blood without RBCs on microscopic examination); prothrombin time; LP if febrile; and a CT scan if symptoms were not explained by laboratory results.

Comparators: None.

Outcomes: A medical condition appeared to be related to the presenting symptoms in 63 of the 100 patients. The medical history was significant in 27, physical examination in 6, alcohol and drug screen in 28, CBC in 5, SMA-7 in 10, CPK in 6, LP in 3, and CT in 8. A greater proportion of individuals had abnormalities noted on these tests that were not judged to be clinically significant or relevant to the etiology of the psychiatric presentation.

Timing: Assessment occurred after arrival at an emergency department.

Setting: Adult emergency department in an urban, county hospital.

Study design: Cohort study.

Study sponsorship: Not described.

Overall risk of study bias: **Medium**

- **Selection bias:** *Low Risk:* The authors used logbook of emergency department patients to identify consecutive patients.
- **Performance bias:** *Low Risk:* The assessments were performed consistently with the entire study population.
- **Attrition bias:** *Low Risk:* Study was retrospective and cross-sectional, so there were no problems with dropouts.
- **Detection bias:** *High Risk:* Determining the relationship between a test result and a patient's psychiatric presentation is a subjective clinical judgment that could be biased by investigators' hypotheses.
- **Reporting bias:** *Low Risk:* The battery of tests was prespecified.
- **Sponsor-related bias:** *Low Risk:* Sponsorship is unclear, but the study was not a pharmaceutical or device-related trial.

Applicability: The patient population constitutes a relatively small proportion of individuals who present to a psychiatric emergency service. Individuals presenting for outpatient treatment are likely to have a very different set of risk factors for medical conditions. The age of the study may also limit its applicability in terms of changes in the healthcare delivery system, laboratory assessments, and the typical characteristics of individuals who present for an emergency evaluation.

Citation: Bartsch DA, Shern DL, Feinberg LE, et al.: Screening CMHC outpatients for physical illness. *Hospital and Community Psychiatry* **41(7):786–790, 1990**

Population: 175 outpatients from two community mental health centers (CMHCs), one urban and one rural, in Colorado.

Intervention: Health history, review-of-systems questionnaire, physical examination, laboratory tests (urinalysis, SMAC-26 chemistry panel, vitamin B_{12}, folate levels).

Comparators: One control group at each site who did not receive medical screening. The control group at the urban center comprised patients who were not approached for participation in the study. The control group at the rural center comprised patients who were approached but did not participate in the study. The authors explained that there was a smaller number of patients available at the rural center than at the urban center; the proportion of control patients from each center was equal to the proportion of intervention patients from each center.

Outcomes: For the combined sample, 20% had a previously undiagnosed physical health problem, 16% had conditions that could cause or exacerbate their mental disorder, and 46% had physical conditions or laboratory test results that were judged to warrant further medical evaluation.

Timing: Individuals at various stages of outpatient psychiatric treatment assessed between February and May 1985.

Setting: Two CMHCs (one urban and one rural) in Colorado.

Study design: Nonblinded observational study with a comparison "control" group to assess the representativeness of the sample as compared with the clinic population and individuals treated in CMHCs statewide.

Study sponsorship: Unclear; no specific study sponsorship is noted, although study funding is mentioned.

Overall risk of study bias: **High**

- **Selection bias:** *High Risk:* Although individuals were randomly selected for the intervention group at the urban center, all patients at the rural center were asked to participate, and the control group included some individuals who had refused to participate in the intervention group. The fact that the intervention and control groups differed in their characteristics suggests that allocation was not ideal.
- **Performance bias:** *Low Risk:* The assessments were performed consistently with all study participants.
- **Attrition bias:** *High Risk:* A substantial proportion (36%) of individuals who were randomly selected for screening did not participate.
- **Detection bias:** *High Risk:* Judgments about relationship of abnormalities to psychiatric disorder are subjective and potentially influenced by investigators' a priori hypotheses. However, the study did attempt to reduce the risk of bias by using two raters for each determination and calculating the relative rates of agreement between raters.
- **Reporting bias:** *Low Risk:* The battery of tests being used was prespecified.
- **Sponsor-related bias:** *Unclear:* Study funding is mentioned as restricting the sample size, but the funding source is not identified.

Applicability: The patient population reflects individuals attending two CMHCs in Colorado, and demographic characteristics of the sample differ from those of individuals seen at that CMHC and at CMHCs across the state. Individuals presenting for outpatient CMHC treatment in Colorado are likely to have a different set of risk factors for medical conditions than individuals in other states or those presenting to other psychiatric treatment settings. The age of the study may also limit its applicability in terms of changes in the healthcare delivery system, laboratory assessments, and the typical characteristics of individuals who are followed in an outpatient CMHC setting.

Grading of Supporting Body of Research Evidence

Risk of bias: **High Risk:** studies are unblinded and observational, with judgments about the relationship between screening results and medical causes of psychiatric symptoms being a subjective determination and associated with potential for bias.

Consistency: **Consistent:** medical conditions related to psychiatric symptoms were consistently found for a sizeable portion of patients studied.

Directness: **Indirect:** uses intermediate outcomes such as diagnosis rather than patient-specific health benefits. Also, the outcomes are indirectly related to those of the overarching key questions regarding assessment of medical health to improve diagnostic accuracy and treatment safety.

Precision: **Imprecise:** there was prominent variability across study findings, even among studies done in comparable settings of care.

Dose-response relationship: **Not applicable.**

Magnitude of effect: **Not applicable.**

Confounding factors (including likely direction of effect):   Depending on the investigators' a priori hypotheses, the lack of blinding could influence the judgments about contributors to psychiatric symptoms and the clinical significance of laboratory abnormalities. This could produce confounding effects in either direction.

Publication bias: **Not able to be assessed.**

Applicability: The age of the studies range from 18 to 31 years, and the studies were conducted in private outpatient settings, which limits applicability to current treatment methods and other types of settings. Also, the outcomes measured in the studies are not directly related to the outcomes in our key questions. This body of evidence examines the proportion of psychiatric patients who have a medical condition that causes or exacerbates psychiatric symptoms, whereas the outcome of interest is whether assessment of certain aspects of medical health improves diagnostic accuracy and treatment safety.

Overall strength of research evidence: **Low.**

Differences of Opinion in Rating the Strength of Recommendations

There were minor differences of opinion among the members of the work group with respect to assessing aspects of patients' medical health. Some members of the group thought that the potential benefits of assessment of some of the recommended items were closely balanced with the potential harm that might result if crucial aspects of the evaluation of an individual patient go unaddressed, particularly when the evaluation is time constrained. Another concern raised was that assessment of the recommended items might not be important for all patients or necessary to include at the initial evaluation (as compared with follow-up visits). The recommended items for which there was disagreement on the basis of these concerns by one or two group members were as follows: involuntary movements or abnormalities of motor tone; speech, including fluency and articulation; sight and hearing; physical trauma, including head injuries; past or current medical illnesses and related hospitalizations; important past or current treatments or procedures, including complementary and alternative medical treatments; sexual and reproductive history; and past or current sleep abnormalities, including sleep apnea. The work group was unanimous in agreeing to recommend assessment of general appearance and nutritional status, coordination and gait, and allergies or drug sensitivities.

Expert Opinion Survey Results

To what extent do you agree that the initial psychiatric evaluation of any patient should typically (i.e., almost always) include assessment of whether or not the patient has an ongoing relationship with a primary care health professional?

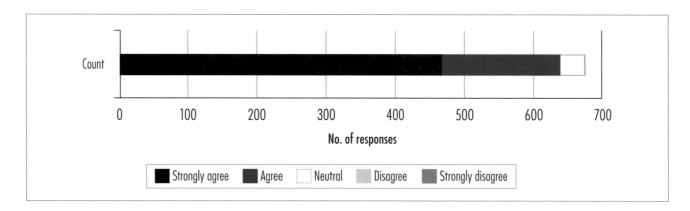

Percentage of experts who "strongly agreed" or "agreed" that the initial psychiatric evaluation of any patient should typically (i.e., almost always) include assessment of whether or not the patient has an ongoing relationship with a primary care health professional: 94.6%.

In your initial psychiatric evaluations, do you typically (i.e., almost always) assess whether or not your patients have an ongoing relationship with a primary care health professional?

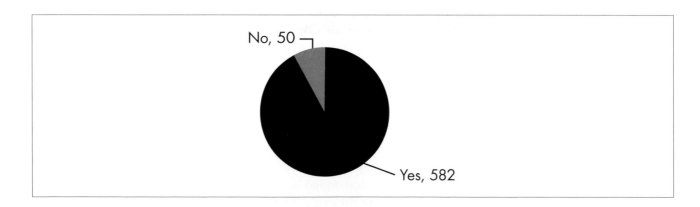

To what extent do you agree that diagnostic accuracy and treatment safety are improved when the initial psychiatric evaluation of any patient typically (i.e., almost always) includes assessment of the following aspects of his or her current general medical status?[6]

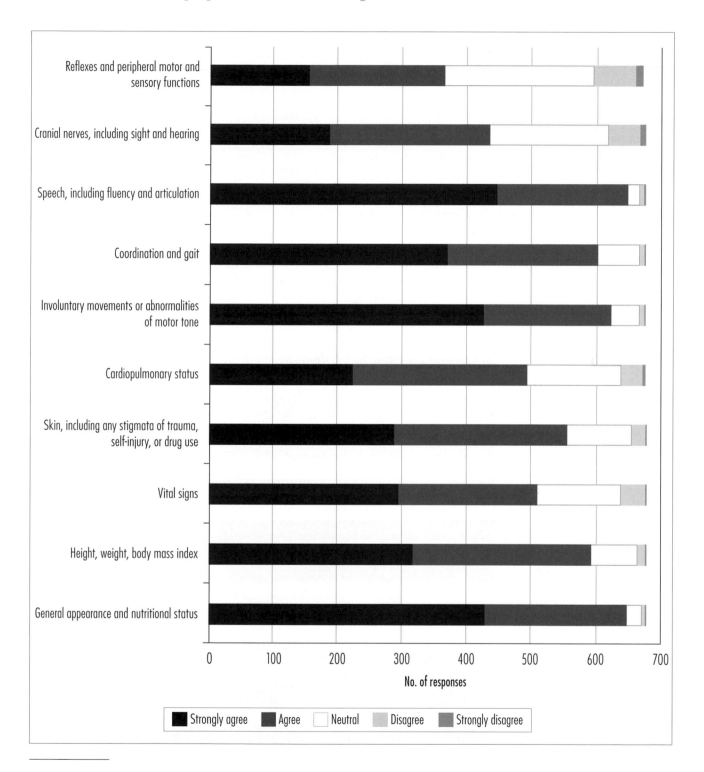

[6] "Assessment" is defined here as a) performing a physical examination on the patient, b) directing another clinician (e.g., a resident) to perform the exam, or c) reviewing the results of a recent physical examination performed by another clinician.

Percentage of experts who "strongly agreed" or "agreed" that diagnostic accuracy and treatment safety are improved when the initial psychiatric evaluation of any patient typically (i.e., almost always) includes assessment of the following aspects of his or her current general medical status:

Reflexes and peripheral motor and sensory functions	54.5%
Cranial nerves, including sight and hearing	64.8%
Speech, including fluency and articulation	96.3%
Coordination and gait	89.2%
Involuntary movements or abnormalities of motor tone	92.4%
Cardiopulmonary status	73.6%
Skin, including any stigmata of trauma, self-injury, or drug use	82.5%
Vital signs	75.6%
Height, weight, BMI	87.9%
General appearance and nutritional status	95.8%

Do you typically (i.e., almost always) assess these items during initial psychiatric evaluations of your patients, either by direct examination or by review of the results of a recent examination by another clinician?

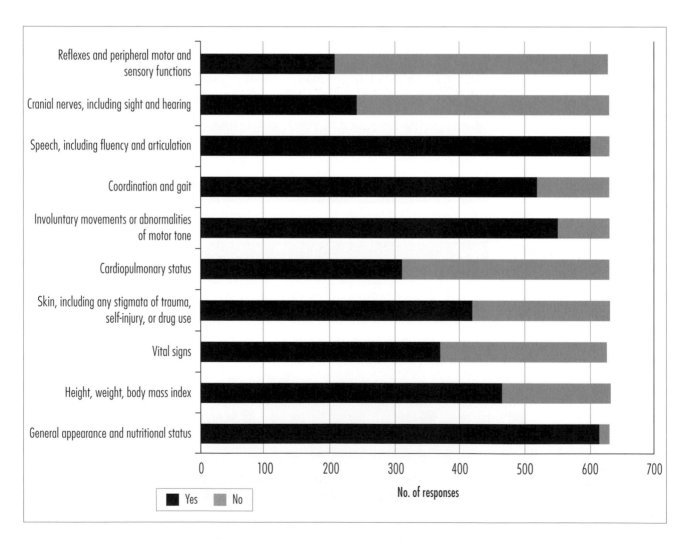

To what extent do you agree that diagnostic accuracy and treatment safety are improved when the initial psychiatric evaluation of any patient typically (i.e., almost always) includes assessment of the following aspects of his or her general medical history? Assessment may occur directly or by review of the results of a recent assessment by another clinician.

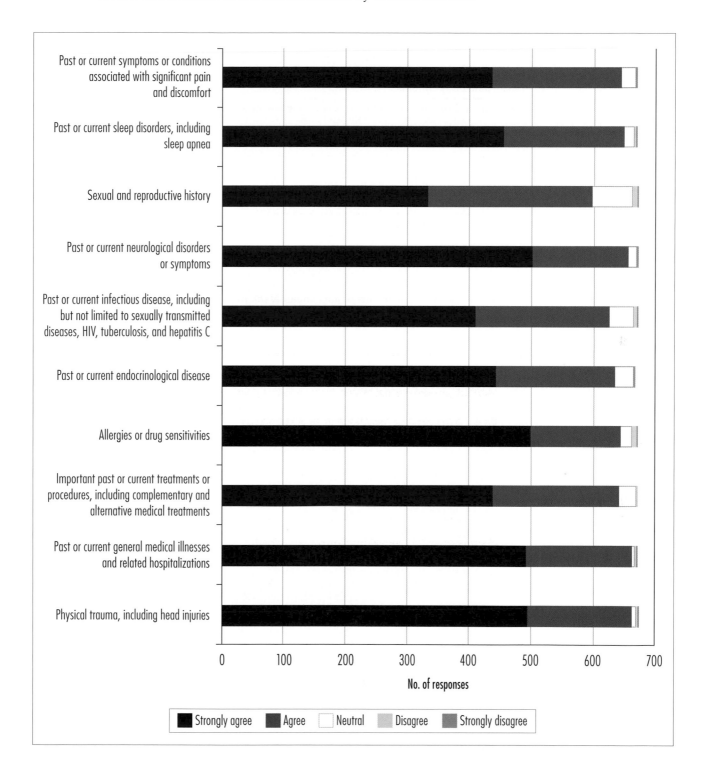

Percentage of experts who "strongly agreed" or "agreed" that diagnostic accuracy and treatment safety are improved when the initial psychiatric evaluation of any patient typically (i.e., almost always) includes assessment of the following aspects of his or her general medical history:[7]

Past or current symptoms or conditions associated with significant pain and discomfort	96.3%
Past or current sleep disorders, including sleep apnea	97.0%
Sexual and reproductive history	89.0%
Past or current neurological disorders or symptoms	97.9%
Past or current infectious disease, including but not limited to sexually transmitted diseases, HIV, tuberculosis, and hepatitis C	93.2%
Past or current endocrinological disease	95.2%
Allergies or drug sensitivities	96.3%
Important past or current treatments or procedures, including complementary and alternative medical treatments	95.4%
Past or current general medical illnesses and related hospitalizations	98.7%
Physical trauma, including head injuries	98.4%

---

[7] Assessment may occur directly or by review of the results of a recent assessment by another clinician.

Do you typically (i.e., almost always) assess these items during initial psychiatric evaluations of your patients?

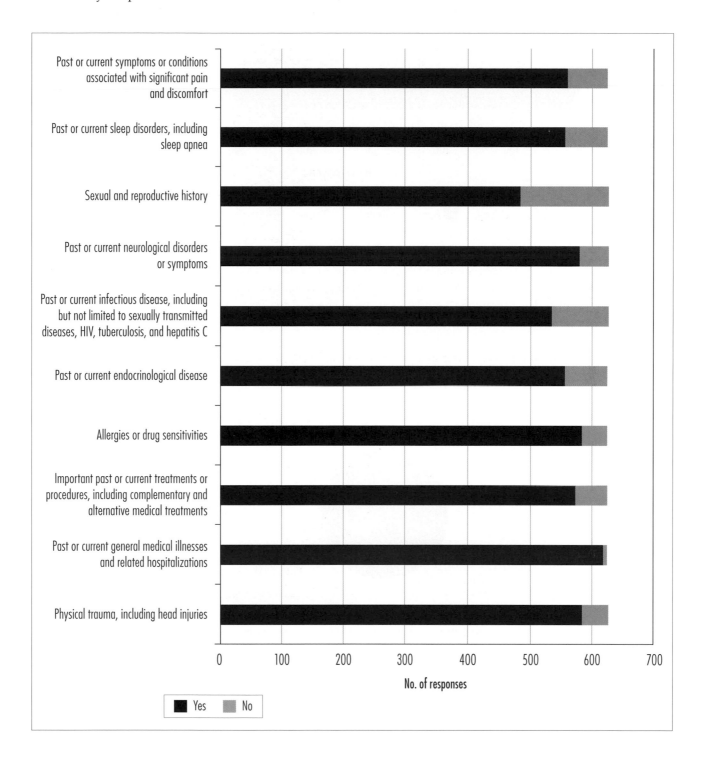

To what extent do you agree that diagnostic accuracy and treatment safety are improved when the initial psychiatric evaluation of any patient typically (i.e., almost always) includes review of all medications he or she is currently or recently taking and the side effects of these medications?[8]

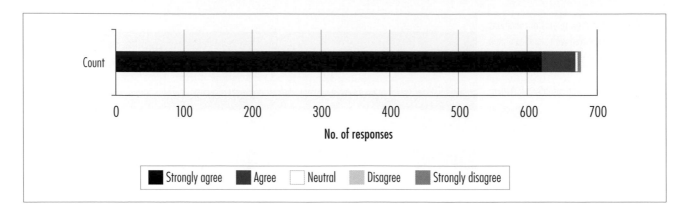

Percentage of experts who "strongly agreed" or "agreed" that diagnostic accuracy and treatment safety are improved when the initial psychiatric evaluation of any patient typically (i.e., almost always) includes review of all medications he or she is currently taking or was recently taking and the side effects of these medications: 99.4%.

During initial psychiatric evaluations, do you typically (i.e., almost always) review all medications your patients are currently or recently taking and the side effects of these medications?

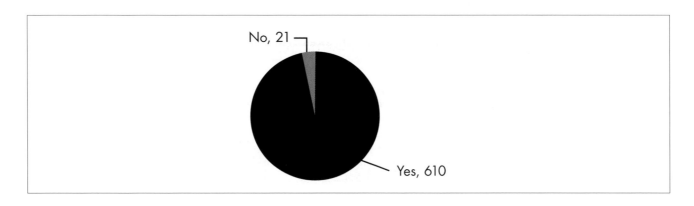

[8] "All medications" means both prescribed and nonprescribed medications, herbal and nutritional supplements, and vitamins.

To what extent do you agree that diagnostic accuracy and treatment safety are improved when the initial psychiatric evaluation of any patient typically (i.e., almost always) includes the following elements of a review of systems?

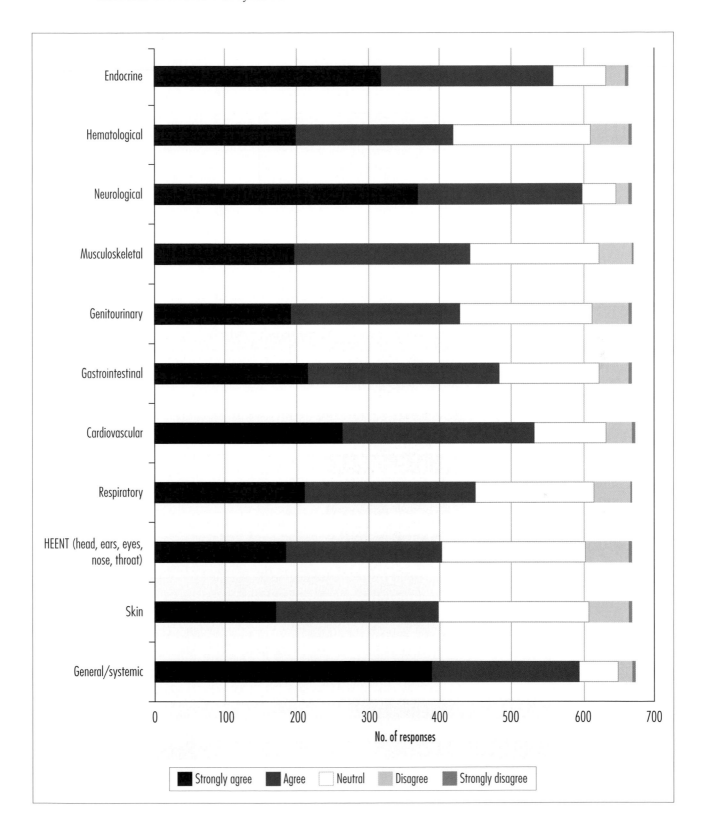

Percentage of experts who "strongly agreed" or "agreed" that diagnostic accuracy and treatment safety are improved when the initial psychiatric evaluation of any patient typically (i.e., almost always) includes the following elements of a review of systems:

Endocrine	84.2%
Hematological	62.7%
Neurological	89.6%
Musculoskeletal	66.1%
Genitourinary	64.3%
Gastrointestinal	72.4%
Cardiovascular	78.9%
Respiratory	67.4%
HEENT (head, ears, eyes, nose, throat)	60.1%
Skin	59.7%
General/systemic	88.6%

Do you typically (i.e., almost always) review these items during initial psychiatric evaluations of your patients?

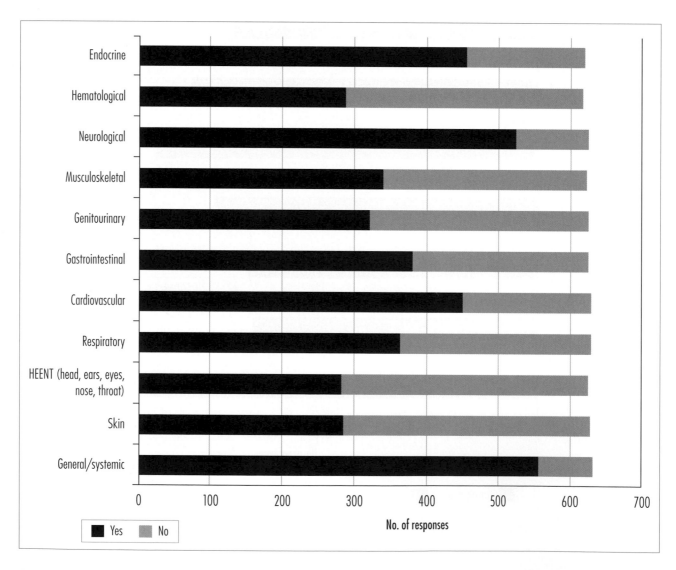

GUIDELINE VII. Quantitative Assessment

Clinical Questions

Development of this guideline was premised on the following clinical questions:

For patients who present with a psychiatric symptom, sign, or syndrome in any setting, is clinical decision making improved when quantitative measures of the following are typically (i.e., almost always) obtained within the scope of the initial psychiatric evaluation, as compared with non-quantitative clinician assessment?[9]

a. **Symptoms**
b. **Level of functioning**
c. **Quality of life**

For patients who present with a psychiatric symptom, sign, or syndrome in any setting, are clinical decision making and treatment outcomes improved when quantitative measures of the following are typically (i.e., almost always) obtained on at least one occasion after the initial psychiatric evaluation, compared to nonquantitative clinician assessment?

a. **Symptoms**
b. **Adverse effects of treatment**
c. **Level of functioning**
d. **Quality of life**

---

[9] "Quantitative measures" are defined as clinician- or patient-administered tests or scales that provide a numerical rating of features such as symptom severity, level of functioning, or quality of life and that have been shown to be valid and reliable.

Review of Supporting Research Evidence

Overview of Studies

Study	Subjects/Method	N	Design/ Duration	Outcomes
van Eijk et al. 2009	Patients admitted to a mixed medical and surgical intensive care unit (ICU) were assessed by trained ICU nurses using the Confusion Assessment Method for the Intensive Care Unit (CAM-ICU) or the Intensive Care Delirium Screening Checklist (ICDSC); by the ICU physician; and by a psychiatrist, geriatrician, or neurologist as a reference rater.	126	Cross-sectional; November 2006–July 2007	The CAM-ICU showed superior sensitivity and negative predictive value (64% and 83%) compared with the ICDSC (43% and 75%). The ICDSC showed higher specificity and positive predictive value (95% and 82% vs. 88% and 72%). As compared with the reference rater, ICU physicians identified delirium with a sensitivity of 29% and specificity of 96%, indicating that ICU physicians underdiagnose delirium.
van den Boogaard 2009	A delirium screening instrument, CAM-ICU, was implemented in a 40-bed ICU. Adoption of the instrument and frequency and duration of haloperidol use were assessed.	641 patients March–June post-CAM-ICU implementation compared with 512 and 589 patients in prior 2 years.	Nonblinded, nonrandomized intervention study; haloperidol use assessed over a 4-month period and compared with 4-month periods in prior 2 years.	Almost two times more patients with delirium were detected with the use of the CAM-ICU. More patients were treated with haloperidol (9.9%–14.8%, $P<0.001$), but with a lower dose (6 mg, from 18 mg; $P=0.01$) and for a shorter time period (3 [interquartile range (IQR): 1–5] days, from 5 [IQR:2–9] days; $P=0.02$).
Thomas et al. 2012	The German version of the Confusion Assessment Method (CAM) was used to identify delirium among individuals admitted to an academic geriatric hospital in Germany.	102	Cross-sectional; October 2003–March 2004.	CAM had a sensitivity of 74% and a specificity of 100% relative to clinical diagnosis using DSM-IV criteria and a sensitivity of 82% and specificity of 91% compared with clinical diagnosis using ICD-10. Adding ratings of psychomotor activity to the CAM approach enhanced specificity but reduced sensitivity.

Grading of Quality of Individual Studies

Citation: van Eijk MM, van Marum RJ, Klijn IA, et al.: Comparison of delirium assessment tools in a mixed intensive care unit. *Critical Care Medicine* **37(6):1881–1885, 2009**

Population: During an 8-month period, 126 patients (mean age=62.4 years, SD=15.0; mean Acute Physiology and Chronic Health Evaluation II score 20.9, SD=7.5) admitted to a 32-bed mixed medical and surgical ICU were studied. Excluded were deeply sedated patients (defined as a Ramsay score>4), comatose patients (defined as a Glasgow Coma Score<8), patients for whom no informed consent was obtained, patients who did not speak or understand Dutch or English, or patients who were deaf.

Intervention: The patients included in the study were assessed independently by trained ICU nurses using either the CAM-ICU or the ICDSC. Furthermore, the ICU physician was asked whether a patient was delirious or not. A psychiatrist, geriatrician, or neurologist serving as a reference rater diagnosed delirium using established criteria.

Comparators: Both the standardized assessment instruments and the ICU physician's impression during standard care were compared with a neuropsychiatric assessment performed by an expert (geriatrician, psychiatrist, or neurologist) who served as a reference rater.

Outcomes: The reference raters identified 34% of the patient sample as having signs and symptoms that met diagnostic criteria for delirium, whereas the CAM-ICU, ICDSC, and ICU physicians identified delirium in 29%, 19%, and 13% of patients, respectively. The CAM-ICU showed superior sensitivity and negative predictive value (64% and 83%) compared with the ICDSC (43% and 75%). The ICDSC showed higher specificity and positive predictive value (95% and 82% vs. 88% and 72%). The sensitivity and specificity of the ICU physicians' clinical impression were 29% and 96%, respectively.

Timing: Study assessments took place during an 8-month period, from November 2006 to July 2007.

Setting: The study was performed in a 32-bed multidisciplinary ICU of the University Medical Center Utrecht, the Netherlands, with adult medical, surgical, neurological, neurosurgical, and cardiothoracic surgical patients.

Study design: Cross-sectional.

Overall risk of study bias: **Moderate**

- **Selection bias:** *Low Risk:* All patients in the ICU were included in the study other than sedated and comatose patients, patients who did not speak English or Dutch, and deaf patients. It is unlikely that these exclusion criteria would have introduced bias in the study.
- **Performance bias:** *Moderate Risk:* The delirium evaluations were administered by different investigators who were blinded to each other's assessments, thus limiting the chance of systematic differences in the treatment of the participants. There is a risk of co-interventions, because medical treatment while in the ICU was not controlled. Some patients received psychotropic medications between evaluations; the study investigators analyzed these patients separately and did not find any differences from the study population as a whole.
- **Attrition bias:** *Not applicable.*
- **Detection bias:** *Moderate Risk:* The reference assessment was used as a gold standard, and depending on the training and experience of the raters, there could be detection bias in this reference. There was no attempt to verify these reference assessments with a second rater. Also, evaluations were not performed at the same time, and because delirium is by nature a fluctuating disorder, a bias in the diagnosing of delirium was possible.
- **Reporting bias:** *Low Risk:* There is no indication of selective outcome reporting.
- **Sponsor-related bias:** *Low Risk:* The authors did not disclose any potential conflicts of interest. The authors were all affiliated with the University Medical Center Utrecht, The Netherlands.

Setting: The study was performed in an academic geriatric center in Heidelberg, Germany, among individuals admitted for a variety of problems, including falls, infections, metabolic disease, cardiovascular or cardiopulmonary conditions, and psychiatric diagnoses with comorbid medical problems.

Study design: Cross-sectional.

Overall risk of study bias: **Moderate**

- **Selection bias:** *Moderate Risk:* Because only patients admitted on Tuesdays or Fridays were included, it is possible that patients admitted on a weekend have different characteristics than those admitted during the week.
- **Performance bias:** *Moderate Risk:* The delirium evaluations were administered by different investigators who were blinded to each other's assessments, thus limiting the chance of systematic differences in the treatment of the participants. There is a risk of co-interventions, because medical treatment while in the unit was not controlled.
- **Attrition bias:** *Not applicable.*
- **Detection bias:** *Moderate Risk:* The reference assessment was used as a gold standard, and depending on the training and experience of the raters, there could be detection bias in this reference. There was no attempt to verify these reference assessments with a second rater. Also, evaluations were not performed at the same time, and because delirium is by nature a fluctuating disorder, a bias in the diagnosing of delirium was possible.
- **Reporting bias:** *Low Risk:* There was no indication of selective outcome reporting.
- **Sponsor-related bias:** *Low Risk:* The authors did not disclose any potential conflicts of interest.

Applicability: This study is limited to the diagnosis of delirium in hospitalized geriatric patients. Also, the assessments were performed by gerontologists, psychologists, and physicians in training rather than by psychiatrists.

Grading of Supporting Body of Research Evidence

Risk of bias: **High:** The body of evidence is made up of only observational studies of varying quality.

Consistency: **Consistent:** All studies used a quantitative assessment tool to aid in diagnosis.

Directness: **Indirect:** Three studies indicate that use of a quantitative measurement improves clinical diagnosis. Diagnostic accuracy is indirectly related to clinical decision making and treatment outcomes.

Precision: **Not applicable.**

Dose-response relationship: **Not applicable.**

Magnitude of effect: **Weak:** Three studies showed that evaluations based on a quantitative assessment are superior to nonquantitative assessments, although one study showed benefit for one specific assessment scale but not another.

Confounding factors (including likely direction of effect): **Absent.**

Applicability: Two of the studies were done in an ICU, and the other study was done in an inpatient geriatric facility. The assessments were performed by nonpsychiatrist health care staff, although quantitative assessment of delirium would be similar to that done by psychiatric consultants. Also, the studies were only about delirium and not about psychiatric symptoms or diagnoses in general.

Overall strength of research evidence: **Low.**

Differences of Opinion in Rating the Strength of Recommendations

Four members of the work group voted to recommend the use of quantitative measures, but the other four members of the group thought that the potential benefits of using measures were uncertain. As a result, a suggestion rather than a recommendation was made.

Expert Opinion Survey Results

To what extent do you agree that clinical decision making is improved when quantitative measures of the following are typically (i.e., almost always) obtained within the scope of the initial psychiatric evaluation of any patient, as compared with nonquantitative clinician assessment?[10]

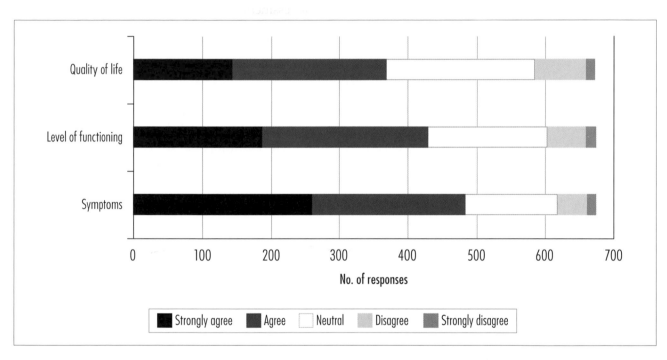

Percentage of experts who "strongly agreed" or "agreed" that clinical decision making is improved when quantitative measures of the following are typically (i.e., almost always) obtained within the scope of the initial psychiatric evaluation of any patient, as compared with nonquantitative clinician assessment:

Quality of life	54.9%
Level of functioning	63.8%
Symptoms	71.7%

---

[10] "Quantitative measures" are defined as clinician- or patient-administered tests or scales that provide a numerical rating of features such as symptom severity, level of functioning, or quality of life and have been shown to be valid and reliable.

Do you typically (i.e., almost always) obtain quantitative measures of these items from your patients within the scope of an initial psychiatric evaluation?

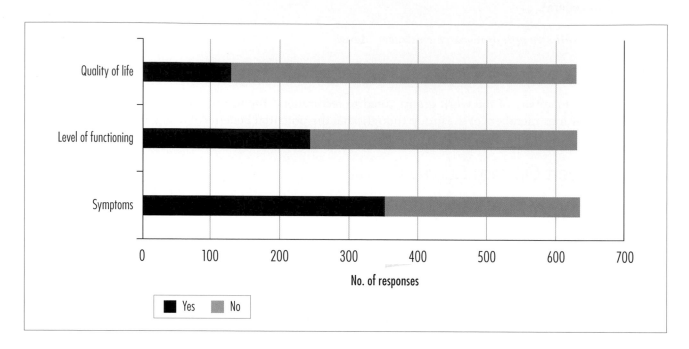

To what extent do you agree that clinical decision making and treatment outcomes are improved when quantitative measures of the following are typically (i.e., almost always) obtained on at least one occasion after the initial psychiatric evaluation of any patient, compared with nonquantitative clinician assessment?

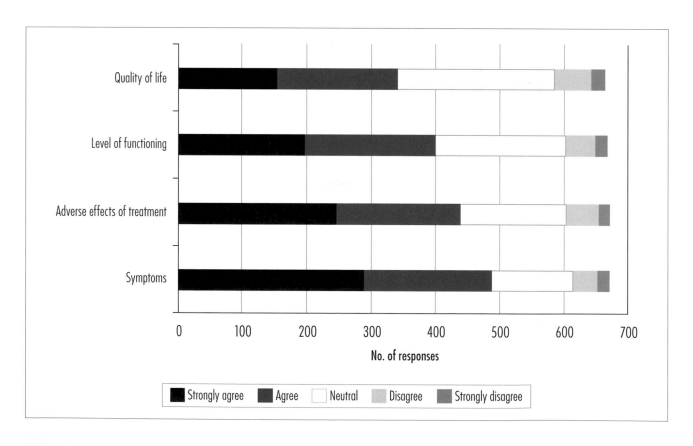

Percentage of experts who "strongly agreed" or "agreed" that clinical decision making and treatment outcomes are improved when quantitative measures of the following are typically (i.e., almost always) obtained on at least one occasion after the initial psychiatric evaluation of any patient, compared with nonquantitative clinician assessment:

Quality of life	51.5%
Level of functioning	60.0%
Adverse effects of treatment	65.4%
Symptoms	72.8%

How frequently do you think these measures should be taken?

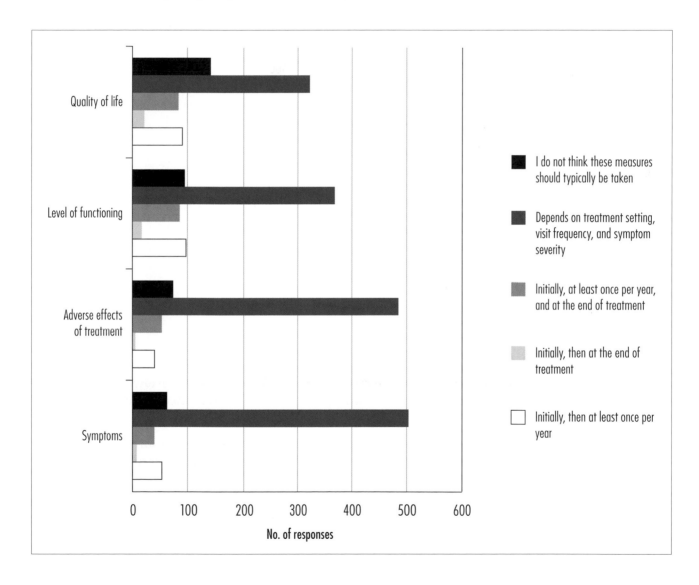

Do you typically (i.e., almost always) obtain quantitative measures of these items on at least one occasion after initial evaluations of your patients?

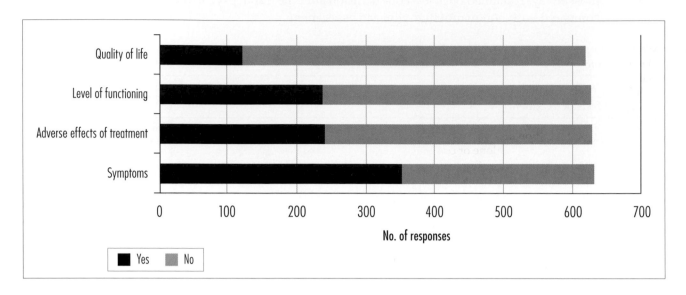

GUIDELINE VIII. Involvement of the Patient in Treatment Decision Making

Clinical Questions

Development of this guideline was premised on the following clinical questions:

For patients who present with a psychiatric symptom, sign, or syndrome in any setting and have the capacity for decision making, are the therapeutic alliance and treatment adherence improved by explaining the following?

a. The diagnosis
b. Risks of untreated illness
c. Treatment options
d. Benefits and risks of treatment

For patients who present with a psychiatric symptom, sign, or syndrome in any setting and have the capacity for decision making, are the therapeutic alliance and treatment adherence improved by asking about treatment-related preferences?

For patients who present with a psychiatric symptom, sign, or syndrome in any setting and have the capacity for decision making, are the following improved by "shared decision making"?[11]

a. Treatment adherence
b. Therapeutic alliance
c. Clinician satisfaction
d. Patient satisfaction

_____

[11] "Shared decision making" is defined as collaboration between clinicians and patients about decisions pertinent to treatment, when the patient has capacity for decision making.

Review of Supporting Research Evidence

Overview of Studies

Study	Subjects/Method	N	Design/ Duration	Outcomes
Buchkremer et al. 1997	Outpatients with schizophrenia were randomly assigned to receive psychoeducational medication management training (PMT) alone or combined with cognitive psychotherapy (CP) and/or key-person counseling (KC), and compared with a nonspecifically treated control group.	191	Randomized, controlled, nonblinded intervention study; 132 subjects assessed at 2 years post-treatments (intention-to-treat used).	The PMT+CP+KP group had a significant reduction in rehospitalization rates compared with control subjects. The relapse rate in all treatment groups was lower than in the nonspecifically treated control group, but there were no statistically significant differences among the treatment groups. Because psychoeducation was included in all treatment groups, this intervention may help with lowering relapse.
Wilder et al. 2010	Patients with severe mental illness recorded medication preferences in advanced directives. Authors compared prescribed medications with patient preferences.	123	Randomized, nonblinded intervention study; 12 months.	Patients requested a median of two medications, and refused a median of one medication, on advanced directives. There was a 27% increase in the number of requested medications prescribed after 12 months. Receiving at least one requested medication predicted higher adherence.
Degmecić et al. 2007	Inpatients with schizophrenia were educated about the illness and treatment, then compared with control subjects at admission, discharge, and 3 months postdischarge. Groups were rated for adherence, attitudes toward treatment, symptoms, and social functioning.	60 (30 in education group and 30 control subjects)	Nonrandomized, non-blinded intervention study; assessments on admission to hospital, at discharge, at and 3 months postdischarge.	Authors concluded that education improves adherence and attitudes toward pharmacotherapy. More specific results are unavailable for review.

Study	Subjects/Method	N	Design/ Duration	Outcomes
Pitschel-Walz et al. 2006	Inpatients with schizophrenia and schizoaffective disorder were randomly assigned to a psychoeducational intervention or a control group. The intervention consisted of 8 sessions for patients and 8 sessions for their relatives.	236	Randomized intervention study; 4- to 5-month intervention with assessments at 12 and 24 months.	Intervention group had significantly lower rehospitalization rates at 12 and 24 months and had better compliance. The authors concluded that a relatively brief intervention of eight psychoeducational sessions with systematic family involvement in simultaneous groups can considerably improve the treatment of schizophrenia.
Gray 2000	Outpatients taking clozapine were randomly assigned to three sessions of patient education or a control group of standard care.	44 (22 in intervention group and 22 in control group).	Randomized, single-blind intervention study; assessments at baseline and at 5 weeks postintervention.	No significant difference found on Drug Attitude Inventory or on the insight scale. Results did not support the hypothesis that brief patient education would be superior to standard of care; it would therefore be unlikely to improve adherence.
Hamann et al. 2006	Inpatients with schizophrenia in 12 hospital wards were randomly assigned either to a shared decision-making intervention or to a control group. Participants in the intervention group were given psychoeducational material, completed a booklet, and participated in treatment planning meetings.	107 (49 in intervention group and 58 in the control group)	Cluster-randomized, controlled, nonblinded intervention study; data collected on admission and at discharge.	Patients in the intervention group reported significantly greater sense of involvement in medical decisions after the initial planning talk, but this difference was not found at discharge. There was no difference in overall satisfaction with treatment, but there was a statistical trend for more positive attitudes about medication in the intervention group, and doctors in this group were more satisfied with overall treatment results.
Hamann et al. 2007	Inpatients with schizophrenia were randomly assigned to a shared decision making group or a control group. The intervention group received psychoeducational material and a planning talk between patient and physician.	107	Cluster-randomized, controlled, nonblinded intervention study; assessments at 6 months and 18 months postdischarge.	No significant differences were found in any outcome measure, but multivariate analysis showed that the intervention group had a positive statistical trend for fewer rehospitalizations, but there was no clear beneficial effect on long-term compliance.

Study	Subjects/Method	N	Design/ Duration	Outcomes
Hornung et al. 1998	Outpatients with schizophrenia were randomly assigned to receive control versus PMT alone or in combination with CP and/or KC.	191 (32 in PMT group, 34 in PMT+CP, 35 in PMT+KC, 33 in PMT+CP+ KC; 57 control subjects)	Randomized, controlled, nonblinded intervention study; assessments at baseline, after intervention, and at 1-year follow-up.	Psychoeducation improved patient attitudes toward treatment, including reduced fear of side effects and more confidence in their medication and physician, but there was no significant difference in compliance at 1-year follow-up. Intervention had no effect on medication management.
Hornung et al. 1996	Outpatients with schizophrenia randomly assigned to control versus PMT alone or in combination with CP and/or KC.	191 (32 in PMT group, 34 in PMT+CP, 35 in PMT+KC, 33 in PMT+CP+ KC; 57 control subjects)	Randomized, controlled, nonblinded intervention study; assessments at baseline, after intervention, and at 1-year follow-up.	Medication compliance increased in both groups but was greater in the training group vs. controls. There was no significant difference in patients' satisfaction of their knowledge of medication, but more patients in the training group did not feel capable of dosing their own medications after the intervention.
Iacoviello et al. 2007	Patients with major depressive disorder were asked what treatment they preferred, then randomly assigned to receive supportive-expressive psychotherapy (PT), sertraline (S), or pill-placebo (P).	75 (Of the 39 preferring psychotherapy: 17 received PT, 12 S, and 10 P; of the 36 preferring medication, 8 received PT, 15 S, and 13 P.)	Randomized, controlled trial; assessments before treatment and during third, fifth, and ninth weeks of treatment.	Among patients who preferred psychotherapy, therapeutic alliance showed positive development over the course of the study if treatment was congruent with the patients' preferences, whereas patients who received a treatment incongruent with their preference showed a decrease in alliance over time. Patients who preferred pharmacotherapy showed no differences regardless of treatment.

Study	Subjects/Method	N	Design/Duration	Outcomes
Merinder et al. 1999	Patients with schizophrenia were randomly assigned to receive an 8-session educational intervention or standard care. The patients' relatives were also invited to participate, though not all subjects had relatives involved.	46 (23 in intervention group, 23 in control group)	Randomized, nonblinded intervention study; 8 weeks of educational sessions, with assessments at baseline, after the intervention, and 1 year post-intervention.	A statistically significant increase in knowledge of schizophrenia in both relatives and patients was demonstrated after the intervention, with a non-significant trend for increased knowledge at 1-year follow-up. Patients and relatives were more satisfied with relatives' involvement in the intervention group. There was a tendency for an increased time to relapse and improvements in symptoms in the intervention group. No differences were found between the groups regarding compliance, insight into psychosis, or Global Assessment of Functioning score, or in relatives' expressed emotion scores, after the intervention or at 1-year follow-up.
Mundt et al. 2001	Outpatients with major depressive disorder receiving antidepressant pharmacotherapy were randomly assigned to receive, or not receive, psychoeducational materials by mail (RHYTHMS program). Patients were then paid to provide self-evaluations of response and satisfaction with treatment, and their prescription records were analyzed for medication compliance.	246	Randomized, nonblinded intervention study; May 1997–August 1998, with assessments at baseline, 4, 12, and 30 weeks.	Patients in the control group initially responded better than those in the intervention group, but this trend did not last. Treatment did not affect the duration of compliance.

Study	Subjects/Method	N	Design/ Duration	Outcomes
Myers and Branth- waite 1992	Outpatients with depression were randomly assigned to one of three groups: group A received one dose of medication at night; group B received three doses of medication during the day; group C patients were allowed to choose either A or B above. Compliance, symptoms, and side effects were assessed at 3, 6, 9, and 12 weeks by interrogation and pill count.	89	Randomized clinical trial; 12 weeks, with assessments at 3, 6, 9, and 12 weeks.	Compliance improved in cases when patients were allowed to choose their regimen, but only when they chose the three-times- per-day regimen. Other groups did not experience the same improvement. Compliance decreased over time in all groups. There was no evidence that compliance produced a better therapeutic result.
Robinson et al. 1986–1987	Patients ready for discharge at a state hospital in Ohio were randomly assigned to receive usual care, a 1- to 2-page handout about medications, or the handout plus a review of the information.	150	Randomized, single-blind intervention study; subjects assessed at discharge and at first follow-up appointment postdischarge.	Subjects who received the handout, with or without verbal explanation, showed improvement in under- standing of treatment. Sub- jects who received written information with verbal reinforcement, but not those who received only the handout, were significantly more treatment compliant than the control subjects.
Sterling et al. 1997	Patients seeking treatment for cocaine dependence received either 12 weeks of weekly individual ther- apy (IND) or an intensive 3-hour, three-times-per- week treatment program (INT). Half the subjects ($n=67$) were given their choice of treatment, with 34 choosing IND and 33 choosing INT, and 30 were randomly assigned to each group.	127	Randomized, nonblinded intervention study; 12 weeks of treatment, with 9-month follow-up.	Patients who chose IND dif- fered from those who chose INT only in 2 of 41 compar- isons: number of previous treatment experiences and Addiction Severity Index (ASI) Alcohol composite score. Allowing patients to choose their course of treat- ment did not significantly enhance retention, the pro- portion of appointments kept, or completion of the 12-week intervention.

Study	Subjects/Method	N	Design/Duration	Outcomes
Vandereycken and Vansteenkiste 2009	On a specialized inpatient unit for treatment of eating disorders, patients who underwent a new admission strategy that emphasized patient choice were compared with control patients who were admitted prior to the new strategy.	174 (87 patients in the intervention arm and 87 control patients who were previously admitted)	Quasi-experimental design; retrospective chart review; 2002–2004; admission strategy involved a 5-day introductory period prior to entering treatment.	Provision of choice at the beginning of treatment significantly reduced the number of dropouts during the first weeks of inpatient treatment. No differences between both strategies on later dropout and weight change (in anorexia nervosa patients) during inpatient treatment were found.
Vreeland et al. 2006	Patients with schizophrenia or schizoaffective disorder were randomly assigned to receive either a 24-week comprehensive, modularized, psychoeducational intervention focused on illness management or standard care.	71	Single-blind, randomized controlled trial; 24-week intervention.	Significant improvement in knowledge about schizophrenia and client satisfaction was observed in the intervention group. No changes were observed in symptoms, treatment adherence, or global functioning.

Grading of Quality of Individual Studies

Citation: Buchkremer G, Klingberg S, Holle R, et al.: Psychoeducational psychotherapy for schizophrenic patients and their key relatives or care-givers: results of a 2-year follow-up. *Acta Psychiatrica Scandinavica* **96(6):483–491, 1997**

Population: A total of 191 patients (80 females and 111 males) from the outpatient departments of nine psychiatric hospitals and a number of psychiatric practices were recruited between May 1989 and February 1990. Patients were eligible for inclusion in the study if the following criteria were fulfilled: i) schizophrenia diagnosed according to DSM-III-R (exclusion of schizoaffective disturbances); ii) at least two acute psychotic episodes within the past 5 years; iii) at least 4 weeks of psychopathological stabilization; iv) indication for long-term neuroleptic medication on an outpatient basis; and v) no secondary psychiatric diagnosis. A total of 147 patients took part in the scheduled therapeutic approach, with hospitalization data obtained from 132 of these subjects at the 2-year follow-up. In total, 20% dropped out of the treatment group and 29% of the patients dropped out of the control group.

Intervention: Psychoeducational medication management training (PMT), cognitive psychotherapy (CP) and key-person counseling (KC) were carried out in various combinations.

Comparators: The control group comprised patients undergoing routine care.

Outcomes: In the second follow-up year, all treatment groups had lower but not significantly different relapse rates compared with the control group. The most intensive treatment (PMT + CP + KC) produced a clinically relevant reduction in rehospitalization, with a 24% rate of rehospitalization compared with a rate of 50% in the control group, although the statistical significance of this effect was nominal. When the treatment groups were considered as a whole and compared with patients in the control group, patients who had received any of the interventions showed greater social functioning and confidence in the therapist and medications at the 2-year follow-up but did not differ on measures of rehospitalization, psychopathological symptoms, or medication adherence.

Timing: Patients were recruited from May 1989 to February 1990. The interventions were carried out on different schedules, based on the intervention. The PMT was carried out in 10 sessions (first 5 weekly, second 5 every other week). The CP took place over 15 sessions (7 weekly, 8 every other week). KC was delivered over 20 sessions. Follow-up occurred 2 years after the intervention(s).

Setting: Outpatients from the outpatient departments of nine psychiatric hospitals and a number of psychiatric practices in Germany.

Study design: Randomized, controlled, nonblinded intervention study.

Overall risk of study bias: **Low**

- **Selection bias:**   *Low Risk:* The exclusion criteria do not appear to introduce bias, and patients were randomly assigned to the various treatment arms (or control group).
- **Performance bias:**   *Low Risk:* There is no evidence of systematic differences in the treatment of patients or of protocol deviation.
- **Attrition bias:**   *Moderate Risk:* An intention-to-treat analysis was used for dropouts, which constituted 20%–30% of participants. However, patients who drop out may be more likely to be rehospitalized (e.g. if the subject dropped out because of worsening symptoms).
- **Detection bias:**   *Low Risk:* The authors noted that rehospitalization data were obtained directly from the institution, with patient consent.
- **Reporting bias:**   *Low Risk:* There is no evidence of selective outcome reporting.
- **Sponsor-related bias:**   *Low Risk:* There is no conflict of interest statement in the study. This study was funded by the German Ministry of Research and Technology.
- **Applicability:**   This study measured rehospitalization rates as a proxy for overall clinical outcome. However, the clinical question is concerned with whether education improves adherence, alliance, and satisfaction. Participants had a diagnosis of schizophrenia and received treatment in an outpatient setting, which limits applicability to other diagnoses and settings. Also, the study population is German, which limits applicability to patients in the United States.

Citation: Wilder CM, Elbogen EB, Moser LL, et al.: Medication preferences and adherence among individuals with severe mental illness and psychiatric advance directives. *Psychiatric Services* **61(4):380–385, 2010**

Population: Participants were outpatients receiving community-based treatment in one of two county-based programs who were 18–65 years old and had a chart diagnosis of schizophrenia, schizoaffective disorder, bipolar disorder with psychotic features, or major depressive disorder with psychotic features. Eighty-three percent of participants (*n*=390) were randomly drawn from de-identified client lists of the two mental health programs that had been prescreened for eligibility. The remaining 17% of participants (*n*=79) were randomly assigned after being identified from sequential admissions from the mental health programs to the regional state hospital with the goal of increasing the proportion of individuals with severe mental illness and potential decisional incapacity.

Intervention: A total of 123 persons with severe mental illness recorded medication preferences in psychiatric advance directives and were reassessed after 12 months of follow-up. The intervention was adapted from several medical and psychiatric advance directive planning tools and included an approximately 2-hour, semistructured, manualized interview and guided discussion of choices for planning mental health care during future periods of incapacity. The facilitator also assisted participants in completing legal psychiatric advance directive documents, obtaining witnesses, getting documents notarized, and filing forms in the medical record and electronic registry.

Comparators: The control group was provided with general information about psychiatric advance directives, copies of standard psychiatric advance directive forms, and a toll-free number for the local consumer organization that provides consultation on psychiatric advance directives.

Outcomes: The authors compared patients' stated medication preferences in advanced directives with prescribed medications over 12 months, determined concordance between preferred and prescribed medications, and examined the effect of concordance on medication adherence at 12 months. Participants requested a median of two medications in their psychiatric advance directives (range: 0–6) and refused a median of one medication (range: 0–10). Between baseline and follow-up there was a 27% increase in the number of medications prescribed that had been requested on the psychiatric advance directive (Wilcoxon matched pairs, $P<0.001$). After correction for the number of medications listed in the psychiatric advance directive, a 10% increase in concordance remained significant ($P<0.001$). Being prescribed at least one medication requested in the psychiatric advance directive predicted higher medication adherence at 12 months, after the analysis controlled for relevant covariates (odds ratio=7.8, 95% confidence interval=1.8–34.0).

Timing: Twelve-month follow-up period after intervention. Follow-up interviews were conducted between October 2004 and September 2006.

Setting: Community-based treatment in one of two county-based programs in North Carolina.

Study design: Randomized, nonblinded intervention study.

Overall risk of study bias: **Moderate**

- **Selection bias:** *Low Risk:* The exclusion criteria do not appear to introduce bias, and patients were randomly assigned to the intervention or control group. The sample intentionally overrepresented individuals with severe mental illness.
- **Performance bias:** *Low Risk:* There is no evidence of systematic differences in treatment or co-interventions.
- **Attrition bias:** *Moderate Risk:* Of the 143 who completed an advanced directive, 123 completed a follow-up interview after 1 year. Those who completed the interview may have been more likely to be adherent to medication than those who did not, which would introduce bias. No intention-to-treat analysis was done.
- **Detection bias:** *High Risk:* Patients were interviewed about their adherence, and previous studies have documented that patients tend to overestimate their adherence to medications.
- **Reporting bias:** *Low Risk:* There is no evidence of selective outcome reporting.
- **Sponsor-related bias:** *Low Risk:* This study was funded by grants from the National Institutes of Health and by the John D. and Catherine T. MacArthur Foundation. The authors, Dr. Swanson and Dr. Swartz, have received research support from Eli Lilly. Dr. Swartz has also received consulting and educational fees from AstraZeneca, Bristol-Myers Squibb, Eli Lilly, and Pfizer. The other authors reported no competing interests.

Applicability: This study is applicable to the clinical question, because it seeks to assess adherence to medications when patients participate in their treatment by completing advanced directives. Also, only individuals in outpatient settings who had psychosis as part of their illness were included, which limits applicability to other diagnoses and settings.

Citation: Degmecić D, Pozgain I, Filaković P: Psychoeducation and compliance in the treatment of patients with schizophrenia. *Collegium Antropologicum* 31(4):1111–1115, 2007

Population: Hospitalized patients with schizophrenia at the University Department of Psychiatry in the University Hospital Osijek, Croatia.

Intervention: Thirty patients participated in an education program about schizophrenia, while 30 other patients did not receive this education. Psychoeducation groups were held by a psychiatrist once a week for 1 hour, and patients were educated about the early recognition of schizophrenia symptoms, about the prevention of recurrence of psychotic episodes, about the role of medication in the treatment of schizophrenia, and also about side effects of those medications. Groups consisted of six to eight patients, and on average patients attended four groups. Patients were assessed on admission to the hospital, at discharge, and 3 months after discharge. Assessments included the Brief Psychiatric Rating Scale (BPRS), Compliance Assessment Inventory, Drug Attitude Inventory, Global Assessment of Functioning (GAF), and a 12-item questionnaire about knowledge of the illness.

Comparators: Patients who participated in the educational program were compared with those who did not.

Outcomes: There were statistically significant improvements in schizophrenia symptoms in the intervention group at discharge and 3 months postdischarge based on both the BPRS and GAF. There were also statistically significant improvements in compliance and knowledge of the illness in the intervention group as compared with the control group.

Timing: Inpatients attended, on average, four 1-hour groups and were assessed at admission, discharge, and 3 months postdischarge. Average length of stay was about 4 weeks.

Setting: Inpatient psychiatric service in Croatia.

Study design: Nonrandomized, nonblinded intervention study.

Overall risk of study bias: **High**

- **Selection bias:** *High Risk:* The authors do not state that patients were randomly assigned to the two groups, and they also do not discuss inclusion or exclusion criteria. The authors do state that there were no significant differences in the groups at baseline in any of the core measures. Nevertheless, there could be selection bias without randomization and without a more defined inclusion and exclusion process.
- **Performance bias:** *High Risk:* The intervention involved weekly 1-hour group sessions with a psychiatrist in an inpatient setting. There may be other reasons that patients in the intervention group improved on all the core measures beyond simply receiving education about schizophrenia (e.g., spending more time with the psychiatrist, socializing with other patients). Patients were not blinded in this study, and so those who had been part of the weekly psychoeducational groups may have been more motivated to report that they were compliant or had fewer symptoms by virtue of being in the study.
- **Attrition bias:** *Low Risk:* Attrition was not discussed in the study, implying that all 60 patients initially chosen to be a part of the study also participated in the follow-up.
- **Detection bias:** *High Risk:* All measurements were based on patient self-report, which tends to overestimate adherence. Patient recall of symptoms may also be inaccurate.
- **Reporting bias:** *Low Risk:* There is no evidence of selective outcome reporting.
- **Sponsor-related bias:** *Unknown Risk.* Statements of conflict of interest were not included.

Applicability: This study does measure adherence after educating patients and is thus applicable to the clinical question. However, because of possible unintended interventions discussed in the subsection on performance bias above, it is difficult to conclude that study effects resulted from the intended intervention (i.e., psychoeducation). Also, the patients were diagnosed with schizophrenia and treated in an inpatient unit in Croatia, which limits applicability of the findings to patients in the United States with other diagnoses and in other treatment settings.

Citation: Pitschel-Walz G, Bäuml J, Bender W, et al.: Psychoeducation and compliance in the treatment of schizophrenia: results of the Munich Psychosis Information Project Study. *Journal of Clinical Psychiatry* **67(3):443–452, 2006**

Population: The study population comprised 236 inpatients whose symptoms met DSM-III-R criteria for schizophrenia or schizoaffective disorder and who had regular contact with at least 1 relative or other key person. Inclusion criteria included a diagnosis of schizophrenia or schizoaffective disorder (according to DSM-III-R/ICD-9 criteria), ages 18–65 years, willingness to receive at least 1 year of outpatient treatment, indication for at least a 12-month antipsychotic relapse prevention, and willingness to involve one key person. Exclusion criteria included a distance between the patient's home and the hospital of more than 150 km, no regular contact with relatives, regular substance use within 6 months prior to admission, pregnancy, an IQ of less than 80, lack of competence in German, and no remission in the past 2 years.

Intervention: Patients were randomly assigned to one of two treatment conditions. In the intervention condition, patients and their relatives were encouraged to attend psychoeducational groups over a period of 4–5 months. The patients' and relatives' psychoeducational programs were separate, and each consisted of eight sessions. Patients in the other treatment condition received routine care.

Comparators: Patients and families in the intervention group were compared with control patients who received routine care.

Outcomes: Rates of rehospitalization and medication adherence were assessed at 12 and 24 months. At 12 and 24 months, adherence was better and the rehospitalization rate was significantly reduced ($P<.05$) among patients who attended psychoeducational groups compared with those receiving routine care.

Timing: Outcomes were compared over 12-month and 24-month follow-up periods. The study was conducted from 1990 to 1994.

Setting: Psychiatric State Hospital, Haar, Germany.

Study design: Randomized intervention study.

Overall risk of study bias: **Moderate**

- **Selection bias:** *High Risk:* Randomization was based on "blocks" of 8–12 patients. There is no information on how the patients were divided into the blocks. Inclusion and exclusion criteria included contact with a key person; it is possible that subjects with regular contact with a key person are different from those without such contact (e.g., may have less severe symptoms, stronger social support). Exclusion of subjects with substance use in the previous 6 months means exclusion of a significant subpopulation of patients diagnosed with schizophrenia or schizoaffective disorder, especially if cigarette use was included in the definition of substance use.

- **Performance bias:** *Moderate Risk:* Treating psychiatrists were blind to the randomization. However, the intervention included attendance at group sessions over an extended period of time, which introduces the possibility for unintended interventions (e.g., increased family involvement and interaction with other patients, and increased attention from clinicians).
- **Attrition bias:** *Moderate Risk.* After beginning the study, 26 patients were excluded because of a change in the status of inclusion or exclusion criteria (i.e., change of diagnosis, no indication for antipsychotic relapse prevention, no remission during inpatient stay, and relocation that changed distance between patient's house and hospital). After acceptance into the study but before outpatient treatment began, 16 patients withdrew consent. Thirty-one patients dropped out of the study before the 12-month follow-up. An additional 10 dropped out before the 24-month follow-up. The 41 patients who dropped out may have systematic differences from those who remained in the study; there were no differences in dropout rate between the intervention and control groups.
- **Detection bias:** *Moderate Risk:* Adherence was measured by clinician report and confirmed by plasma drug level measurements. Other outcomes were measured by clinician and patient report.
- **Reporting bias:** *Low Risk:* There is no evidence for selective outcome reporting.
- **Sponsor-related bias:** *Low Risk:* The study was funded by the German Ministry of Research and Technology. The authors reported no conflicts of interest.

Applicability: Patients in this study who were part of the psychoeducational intervention groups, and who had family members participate, did have increased adherence, which is specifically germane to the clinical question. However, this result could be confounded by other benefits of attending groups and having increased family involvement, as discussed in the subsection on performance bias above. Also, the patients were diagnosed with schizophrenia or schizoaffective disorder and treated in inpatient units in Germany, which limits applicability to patients in the United States with other diagnoses and in other treatment settings.

Citation: Gray R: Does patient education enhance compliance with clozapine? A preliminary investigation. *Journal of Psychiatric and Mental Health Nursing* 7(3):285–286, 2000

Population: The study population comprised 44 patients who had been taking clozapine for at least 3 months. Ten patients (4 in the intervention group and 6 in the control group) dropped out of the study.

Intervention: Patients were randomly assigned to receive three sessions, one per week, of patient education ($n=22$) or routine care ($n=22$). The emphasis in the sessions was on discussion about issues and concerns about all therapies the patient was receiving, both pharmacological and psychological, although the focus of much of the discussion was about clozapine. Patients were encouraged to explore the positive and negative aspects of their current and prior treatments.

Comparators: Patients who participated in the educational intervention were compared with those who received routine care.

Outcomes: Patients were assessed at baseline, and again after 5 weeks, using two self-report instruments: the Drug Attitude Inventory and a 10-item insight scale. At 5-week follow up, there were no significant differences between groups in scores on the Drug Attitude Inventory or the insight scale.

Timing: Patients were assessed at baseline and again at 5 weeks. The sessions lasted 3 weeks.

Setting: The sessions occurred in a room on a hospital ward. The research was done in the United Kingdom. The article does not specify whether the patients themselves were inpatients or whether the study sessions were simply performed in the hospital ward.

Study design: Randomized, single-blind intervention study.

Overall risk of study bias: **Moderate**

- **Selection bias:** *Moderate Risk:* There is no description of inclusion or exclusion criteria, other than patients had to have been taking clozapine for at least 3 months. There was mention in the study that the two groups were not different on the core measures at baseline.
- **Performance bias:** *Low Risk:* There were no differences reported in the two treatment groups.
- **Attrition bias:** *Moderate Risk:* Ten patients out of 44 recruited dropped out of the study, and there was no intention-to-treat analysis. Patients who dropped out may have had different responses to the Drug Attitude Inventory and insight scale.
- **Detection bias:** *Moderate Risk:* Patients were assessed using self-reports. This introduces bias, because patients may not accurately report their own attitudes in an effort to give "correct" answers.
- **Reporting bias:** *Low Risk:* There is no evidence of selective outcome reporting.
- **Sponsor-related bias:** *Unknown Risk:* There is no discussion of conflicts of interest or sponsorship.

Applicability: This study focused on a narrow population of patients who had been taking clozapine for the past 3 months. A brief educational intervention did not improve attitudes or insight, but there was no mention of adherence, alliance, or satisfaction with treatment, which were the foci of the clinical question.

Citation: Hamann J, Langer B, Winkler V, et al.: Shared decision making for in-patients with schizophrenia. *Acta Psychiatrica Scandinavica* 114(4):265–273, 2006

Population: Inpatients ages 18–65 years with an ICD-10 diagnosis of schizophrenia or schizophreniform disorder who were fluent in German and willing to give informed consent were included. Exclusion criteria were severe mental retardation, severe psychosis, or short hospital stays that precluded participation. Of the 301 patients with a diagnosis of schizophrenia who were screened during the enrollment period, 107 patients completed the inpatient phase of the trial, with 49 patients receiving the intervention and 58 in the control group.

Intervention: Patients in the intervention group received a 16-page booklet covering the pros and cons of oral versus depot formulation of antipsychotic, first- versus second-generation antipsychotics, psychoeducation, and types of sociotherapeutic intervention. Nurses were instructed in the use of the decision aid and assisted all patients in working through the booklet. Patients met their physicians within 24 hours after having worked through the shared decision-making aid with their nurse.

Comparators: Inpatients who received the shared decision-making intervention were compared with control patients who received routine care.

Outcomes: Patients filled out five different questionnaires, and physicians and nurses also provided information on their perceptions of the patients' performance in using the decision-making aid and planning care. Patients in the intervention group had a better knowledge about their disease ($P=0.01$) and a higher perceived involvement in medical decisions ($P=0.03$) before hospital discharge. Patients in the intervention group were more likely to receive psychoeducation ($P=0.003$). Overall satisfaction with treatment did not differ between patients in the intervention group and the control group. Therapeutic alliance, measured from the clinician's perspective, did not differ between the intervention and control groups. Clinician-rated patient compliance also did not differ between the groups. However, clinicians in the intervention group were more satisfied with treatment achievements than those in the control group. The authors also noted that the intervention was feasible for most of the patients and did not require additional time spent by physicians.

Timing: The intervention took place while patients were in the hospital. Patients were followed for 18 months postdischarge, although the data reported in this paper derive from the comparisons made at the time of hospital discharge. Patients were recruited between February 2003 and January 2004.

Setting: Twelve acute psychiatric wards of two German state hospitals (Bezirkskrankenhaus Haar, Klinikum Agatharied) in the greater Munich area.

Study design: Cluster-randomized, controlled, nonblinded intervention study.

Overall risk of study bias: **Moderate**

- **Selection bias:** *High Risk:* Patients in the intervention group were different in several ways from patients in the control group. Patients in the intervention group had been hospitalized about a week longer during their present stay than patients in the control group; and Positive and Negative Syndrome Scale (PANSS) ratings for positive symptoms were, accordingly, lower in the intervention group. Patients in the intervention group were slightly younger (mean=35.5 years vs. 39.6 years) and had better knowledge about their disease. There were more patients in the intervention group who had been hospitalized involuntarily.
- **Performance bias:** *Moderate Risk:* Patient's self-report measures could have been influenced by the knowledge that they had been in the intervention group.
- **Attrition bias:** *Moderate Risk:* Six patients dropped out of the study (all of whom withdrew consent): five in the intervention group and one in the control group.
- **Detection bias:** *Low Risk:* Much of the data was obtained through the report of multiple individuals (patients, nurses, and psychiatrists), so the ratings were likely adequate in detecting the outcome measures.
- **Reporting bias:** *Low Risk:* There is no evidence of selective outcome reporting.
- **Sponsor-related bias:** *Low Risk:* The trial was funded by the German Ministry of Health and Social Security. There is no evidence of bias by the sponsors.

Applicability: This study is relevant to the clinical question, although it studies a narrow population of patients (inpatients in a German state hospital with a diagnosis of schizophrenia).

Citation: Hamann J, Cohen R, Leucht S, et al.: Shared decision making and long-term outcome in schizophrenia treatment. *Journal of Clinical Psychiatry* 68(7):992–997, 2007

Population: The study population comprised 107 state psychiatric hospital inpatients with a diagnosis of schizophrenia. Additional details on the study population are described in Hamann et al. 2006 (see above).

Intervention: A shared decision-making (SDM) program on antipsychotic drug choice consisting of a decision aid and a planning talk between patient and physician was compared with routine care.

Comparators: Inpatients who received the SDM were compared with control patients, who received routine care.

Outcomes: On the whole, authors found high rates of noncompliance and rehospitalization. There were no differences in rehospitalization or compliance between the intervention and control groups in the univariate analyses at the 6-month and 18-month follow-ups. However, after confounding factors were controlled for in a multivariate analysis, there was a positive trend ($P=0.08$)

for patients who received the intervention to have fewer rehospitalizations. Additionally, a higher desire of the patient for autonomy and better knowledge at discharge were associated with higher hospitalization rates. Long-term medication compliance was poor for up to 50% of the patients. The SDM intervention had no clear effect on compliance.

Timing: Patients were recruited and received SDM from February 2003 to January 2004. Patients were assessed at 6 and 18 months after the intervention.

Setting: Psychiatric state hospitals in Germany.

Study design: Cluster-randomized, controlled, nonblinded intervention study.

Overall risk of study bias: **Moderate**

- **Selection bias:** *Moderate Risk:* Since randomization was done using a cluster approach in which all patients at a given site were randomly assigned to the same treatment arm, site-specific factors may have produced differences in the intervention and control groups.
- **Performance bias:** *Moderate Risk:* Patients in the intervention group were aware of their randomization status and may have been motivated to give answers on the questionnaires or interviews that they thought were desired by the researchers.
- **Attrition bias:** *Moderate Risk:* Sixteen patients were lost to follow-up at 6 months, and 30 were lost to follow-up at 18 months. Four patients withdrew consent, and 2 patients died within 18 months after discharge. In sum, 6-month follow-up data were available for 80% of the sample, and 18-month follow-up data were available for 66%. The authors report that there were no significant differences in dropout rates in the intervention and control groups. Also, there were no differences between patients who continued the trial and those who dropped out, in terms of age, gender, duration of illness, or PANSS score at discharge.
- **Detection bias:** *Low Risk:* Much of the data was obtained through the report of multiple individuals (patients, nurses and psychiatrists), so the ratings were likely adequate in detecting the outcome measures.
- **Reporting bias:** *Low Risk:* There was no evidence of selective outcome reporting.
- **Sponsor-related bias:** *Low risk.* The study was funded by the German Ministry of Health and Social Security. Study authors reported honoraria and research support from various industry sources.

Applicability: This study is relevant to the clinical question, although it studies a narrow population of patients (inpatients in a German state hospital with diagnosis of schizophrenia).

Citation: Hornung WP, Klingberg S, Feldmann R, et al.: Collaboration with drug treatment by schizophrenic patients with and without psychoeducational training: results of a 1-year follow-up. *Acta Psychiatrica Scandinavica* 97(3):213–219, 1998

Population: The patients were recruited for the study from seven psychiatric centers within a rural region of Germany. The inclusion criteria were as follows: diagnosis of schizophrenia according to DSM-III-R; at least two acute schizophrenic episodes within the past 5 years; registration at an outpatient clinic; need for long-term neuroleptic treatment; and psychopathological stabilization throughout the 4 weeks preceding the study. Patients with diagnoses other than an Axis I diagnosis of schizophrenia were excluded.

Intervention: Patients were randomly assigned to four treatment groups and one control group. The treatment groups contained psychoeducational medication training (PMT) alone ($n=32$) or in combination with cognitive psychotherapy (CP) ($n=34$) and ($n=33$)/or ($n=35$) key-person counseling (KC). The 10 sessions of PMT aimed to provide detailed information about schizophrenia and its treatment and to improve medication management by introducing collaboration between the patient and the psychiatrist in determining medication treatment. Subjects were evaluated at baseline, immediately after treatment, and at 1-year follow-up.

Comparators: The treatment arms were compared with one another and with the control patients who received routine care. Each treatment arm contained the psychoeducational medication training.

Outcomes: The baseline measure of good medication compliance was 76.2% for regular attenders and 69.4% for control patients; the posttreatment measure of good medication compliance was 85.7% for regular attenders and 76.6% for control patients. Although compliance improved in both groups, the difference between the two groups was not significant. At 1-year follow-up, good medication compliance was found in 82.9% of regular attenders and 79.2% of control patients; this difference between the groups was also not significant.

Timing: The PMT lasted 10 weeks, and patients were assessed 1 year after treatment.

Setting: Seven psychiatric centers within a rural region of Germany.

Study design: Randomized, controlled, nonblinded intervention study.

Overall risk of study bias: **Moderate**

- **Selection bias:** *Low Risk:* Patients were randomly assigned to one of the various treatment arms or the control group, and the inclusion and exclusion criteria did not appear to introduce bias.
- **Performance bias:** *Low Risk:* There is no evidence of systematic differences in the treatment of the study groups.
- **Attrition bias:** *High Risk:* Eight of the 84 patients in the treatment group and 11 of the 64 patients in the control group were lost to follow-up. It is not clear, based on this article, whether the analysis accounted for the effects of attrition. Patients who dropped out may have been less likely to be engaged in treatment and may have therefore affected the results of the study if their responses had been included.
- **Detection bias:** *Moderate Risk:* Many of the items assessed were based on patient self-report, including a questionnaire about previous medication management over the past year (particularly the patients' level of compliance). Patients are not likely to have a detailed and accurate memory of prior medication management.
- **Reporting bias:** *Low Risk:* There is no evidence of selective outcome reporting.
- **Sponsor-related bias:** *Low Risk:* The study was funded by the German Ministry of Research and Technology.

Applicability: Patients were chosen from rural clinics in Germany, and all had a diagnosis of schizophrenia. This limits the overall applicability of this study to general U.S. populations. However, the study does investigate the relationship between receiving psychoeducation and subsequent attitudes toward treatment and adherence to treatment.

Citation: Hornung WP, Kieserg A, Feldmann R, Buchkremer G: Psychoeducational training for schizophrenic patients: background, procedure and empirical findings. *Patient Education and Counseling* **29(3):257–268, 1996**

Population: The study included 191 outpatients with chronic schizophrenia (134 in the therapy group and 54 in the control group). They were recruited within seven psychiatric centers in a rural region of Germany. Inclusion criteria were diagnosis of schizophrenia according to DSM-III-R, at least two acute schizophrenic episodes within the last 5 years, attending an outpatient clinic, need for long-term neuroleptic treatment, and psychopathological stabilization within 4 weeks prior to the study. Patients with diagnoses other than schizophrenia were excluded.

Intervention: Patients were randomly assigned to four treatment groups and one control group. The treatment groups contained PMT alone ($n=32$) or in combination with CP ($n=34$) and ($n=33$)/ or ($n=35$) KC. The 10 sessions of PMT aimed to provide detailed information about schizophrenia and its treatment and to improve medication management by introducing collaboration between the patient and the psychiatrist in determining medication treatment.

Comparators: The treatment arms were compared with one another and with controls who received routine care. Each treatment arm contained the psychoeducational medication training.

Outcomes: Patients adherence, knowledge of medications, and ratings of ability to self-manage medications were assessed at baseline, immediately after treatment, and at a 1-year follow-up. At the end of the training program, patients who had attended regularly showed significantly better medication compliance relative to their baseline level of compliance and were less confident in their medication self-management skills. By 1 year follow-up, the positive effects of the intervention had diminished.

Timing: Subjects were assessed at baseline, immediately after the intervention, and at 1-year postintervention.

Setting: Outpatients with schizophrenia, recruited from seven mental health clinics in rural Germany.

Study design: Randomized, controlled, nonblinded intervention study.

Overall risk of study bias: **Moderate**

- **Selection bias:** *Low Risk:* Patients were randomly assigned to the various treatment arms, and the inclusion and exclusion criteria did not appear to introduce bias.
- **Performance bias:** *Low Risk:* There is no evidence of systematic differences in the treatment of the study groups.
- **Attrition bias:** *High Risk:* 8 of the 84 patients in the treatment group, and 11 of the 64 patients in the control group, were lost to follow-up. It is not clear, based on this article, whether the analysis accounted for the effects of attrition. Patients who dropped out may have been less likely to be engaged in treatment and may have therefore affected the results of the study if their responses had been included.
- **Detection bias:** *Moderate Risk:* Many of the items assessed were based on patient self-report, including a questionnaire about previous medication management over the past year (particularly the patients' level of compliance). Patients are not likely to have a detailed and accurate memory of prior medication management.
- **Reporting bias:** *Low Risk:* There was no evidence of selective outcome reporting.
- **Sponsor-related bias:** *Low Risk:* The study was funded by the German Ministry of Research and Technology.

Applicability: Patients were chosen from rural clinics in Germany, and all had a diagnosis of schizophrenia. This limits the overall applicability of this study to general U.S. populations. However, the study does investigate the relationship between receiving psychoeducation and subsequent attitudes toward treatment and adherence to treatment.

Citation: Iacoviello BM, McCarthy KS, Barrett MS, et al.: Treatment preferences affect the therapeutic alliance: implications for randomized controlled trials. *Journal of Consulting and Clinical Psychology* 75(1):194–198, 2007

Population: Data were collected from the first 75 patients enrolled in an ongoing study comparing the efficacy of supportive-expressive (SE) psychotherapy with sertraline or pill-placebo in the treatment of major depressive disorder (MDD). Inclusion criteria were a primary diagnosis of MDD as determined with the Structured Clinical Interview for DSM–IV and the 17-item version of the Hamilton Rating Scale for Depression (a score of ≥ 14). Patients were excluded from participation if they had a current or past history of psychosis, bipolar disorder, or substance dependence in the past 6 months and/or current suicide risk or nonresponse to an adequate trial of sertraline or SE therapy within the last year.

Intervention: Subjects were asked what treatment they preferred and then were randomly assigned to receive supportive-expressive psychotherapy, sertraline, or pill-placebo. Treatment preference, alliance, and depressive symptoms were assessed at baseline and periodically throughout the study.

Comparators: Alliance for patients who received their preferred treatment was compared with alliance for patients who did not receive their preferred treatment.

Outcomes: In patients who preferred psychotherapy, therapeutic alliance showed positive development over the course of the study if treatment was congruent with their preferences, whereas patients who received treatment incongruent with their preference showed a decrease in alliance over time. Patients who preferred pharmacotherapy showed no differences regardless of treatment.

Timing: The psychotherapeutic condition consisted of twice-weekly sessions for 4 weeks, followed by weekly sessions for the next 12 weeks. Patients receiving pharmacotherapy treatment were blind to the treatment they were receiving (sertraline or placebo) and were seen in weekly clinical management sessions with a pharmacotherapist for 16 weeks.

Setting: Outpatient setting in Philadelphia, Pennsylvania.

Study design: Randomized, controlled trial.

Overall risk of study bias: **Moderate**

- **Selection bias:** *High Risk:* This study measured the effect on alliance when patients do not get the treatment they prefer, and yet the subjects all had agreed to be randomly assigned to treatment. Only patients who agreed to this randomization were included, and this may have affected the results of the study. Patients who choose psychotherapy may be systematically different from those who choose pharmacotherapy, which limits the ability to attribute effects on therapeutic alliance purely to congruent/incongruent treatment assignment. Also, the exclusion criteria focused on illness characteristics (e.g., history of psychosis, substance dependence) may have introduced bias into the selected sample of patients.
- **Performance bias:** *Moderate Risk:* Patients receiving pharmacotherapy were blinded to whether they received sertraline or placebo. However, there was no control group (e.g., time and attention control) for the psychotherapy group.
- **Attrition bias:** *High Risk:* An intention-to-treat analysis was performed to minimize attrition bias. Nevertheless, because the study was measuring treatment alliance, there is likely a difference in treatment alliance between those who remained with the study and those who were lost to follow-up.

- **Detection bias:** *Moderate Risk:* Self-report measures were used for treatment preference and therapeutic alliance. Subjects in the study may not have accurately reported their attitudes because they may have been trying to give the "right" answer. Depression severity was rated by blind outcome assessors.
- **Reporting bias:** *Low Risk:* There is no evidence of selective outcome reporting.
- **Sponsor-related bias:** *Low Risk:* This research was supported by a National Institute of Mental Health grant. There is no evidence of sponsor-related bias.

Applicability: The study shows that for outpatients with depression, alliance is improved when patients receive their preferred treatment. This answers the clinical question: involving the patient in the treatment plan improves his or her alliance with the clinician. However, subjects were treated in an outpatient setting in one U.S. city for depression, which limits applicability across treatment settings and diagnoses.

Citation: Merinder LB, Viuff AG, Laugesen HD, et al.: Patient and relative education in community psychiatry: a randomized controlled trial regarding its effectiveness. *Social Psychiatry and Psychiatric Epidemiology* **34(6):287–294, 1999**

Population: Subjects were identified from a local case registry and included all patients ages 18-49 years with a clinical ICD-10 diagnosis of schizophrenia who were in treatment at one of two community psychiatric centers in Denmark. A total of 135 patients fulfilled the inclusion criteria and were invited to participate in the study. Of these, 34% (*n*=46) agreed to participate, 27% declined to participate, and 39% did not respond to the invitation.

Intervention: The experimental group received an eight-session intervention conducted weekly, given separately to both patients and their relatives, using a mainly didactic interactive method focused on topics concerning schizophrenia. The control group received the usual treatment provided in community psychiatry (i.e., psychopharmacological treatment, psychosocial rehabilitation efforts, and, to some extent, supportive psychotherapy).

Comparators: Patients undergoing usual outpatient care were compared with those who had received an 8-week psychoeducational intervention, along with their relatives.

Outcomes: A statistically significant increase in knowledge of schizophrenia in both relatives and patients was demonstrated postintervention, and there was a nonsignificant trend at 1-year follow-up. Statistically significant changes in the Verona Service Satisfaction Scale Scores in the subdimension of satisfaction with relatives' involvement were demonstrated both for patients and relatives post-intervention and for patients at 1-year follow-up. There was a tendency for time-to-relapse to be increased in the intervention group post-intervention and for the schizophrenia subscore of the Brief Psychiatric Rating Scale to be reduced in the intervention group at 1-year follow-up. No differences were found between the groups regarding compliance, insight into psychosis, psychosocial function (GAF), or relatives' expressed emotion scores post-intervention or at 1-year follow-up.

Timing: The intervention was 8 weeks long conducted in 1-week sessions. Patients were assessed at baseline, after the intervention, and at 1-year post-intervention.

Setting: Two community mental health centers in Denmark.

Study design: Randomized, nonblinded intervention study.

Overall risk of study bias: **Moderate**

- **Selection bias:** *Moderate Risk:* Of the pool of patients identified from the case registry, a large portion of them did not respond to the invitation to participate (39%) or declined to participate (27%). There was a statistically significant difference between the participants in the intervention group and the control group: a diagnosis of self-destructive behavior (suicide attempt or self-mutilation) was more common among the participants than among those patients who refused or did not respond. There were nonsignificant trends for the participants to have shorter duration of illness and for fewer to have a previous substance abuse diagnosis or to have experienced a previous compulsory admission. These differences may have affected some of the findings in the study.
- **Performance bias:** *Moderate Risk:* It is not clear whether the intervention was being delivered by clinicians who were also involved in the treatment of the control patients, which could result in unrecognized modifications in the approach to usual treatment.
- **Attrition bias:** *Moderate Risk:* Five patients (10.9%) and two relatives (5.7%) took part in fewer than 50% of the educational sessions. In comparison with the completers, these patients were younger and patient and relative dropouts had a higher initial total satisfaction with services. Eight patients (17.4%; four intervention and four control patients) were partly lost to follow-up of compliance or relapse data, as they were referred to private practitioners for further treatment (*n*=5) or moved to another county (*n*=2). One patient in the control group committed suicide during the follow-up period.
- **Detection bias:** *Moderate Risk:* Several scales were used that had varying levels of reliability and validity reported. However, outcome assessors were blind to treatment allocation.
- **Reporting bias:** *Low Risk:* There is no evidence of selective outcome reporting.
- **Sponsor-related bias:** *Low Risk:* The study was funded in part by Lundbeck A/S, Denmark. There is no indication of sponsor-related bias.

Applicability: This study was only concerned with a single diagnosis, schizophrenia, and so the findings may not apply to a general psychiatric population. Also, it was conducted at community mental health clinics in Denmark, which may differ from the models of care available in the United States. These factors limit applicability, but overall the study does address the clinical question, because it assesses patient adherence after an attempt to introduce psychoeducation (for both patients and their relatives).

Citation: Mundt JC, Clarke GN, Burroughs D, et al.: Effectiveness of antidepressant pharmacotherapy: the impact of medication compliance and patient education. *Depression and Anxiety* 13(1):1–10, 2001

Population: The study population comprised 246 depressed patients, diagnosed and treated at one of three outpatient clinics affiliated with the Kaiser-Permanente Northwest Region (KPNW) healthcare system. Inclusion criteria required 1) DSM-IV diagnosis for current major depression, 2) minimum symptom duration of at least 1 month, 3) prescription of an antidepressant medication during the current office visit, and 4) a Hamilton Depression Rating Scale (Ham-D) score of 18 or greater. Patients were excluded from participation if they 1) were under 18 years old, 2) were planning to move away from the area or change HMOs within 1 year, 3) had received psychotherapy or pharmacotherapy for depression during the 6 months prior to study referral, or 4) did not have access to a touch-tone telephone at their residence.

Intervention: This study was designed to investigate the impact of a time-phased patient education program (RHYTHMS™, developed by Pfizer) on medication compliance and treatment outcomes of primary care patients diagnosed with major depression who had started receiving antidepressant pharmacotherapy. Subjects were randomly assigned to either receive or not receive (usual care) the educational materials by mail.

Comparators: Subjects who received the educational materials were compared with those who did not.

Outcomes: Depression severity and functional impairment affecting patients' quality of life were assessed at baseline and 4, 12, and 30 weeks later. Self-reported impressions of improvement and patient satisfaction with treatment were also assessed at follow-up. Clinical assessment data were obtained using an interactive voice response (IVR) system. Upon study completion, prescription fill data of the subjects were extracted from the KPNW Pharmacy System for analysis of medication compliance. Most of the study subjects (63.5%) had responded to the pharmacotherapy treatment by study end-point. Few statistically significant differences in either treatment outcomes or duration of medication compliance were found between the treatment groups, and significant differences found were of fairly small magnitude. Patients not receiving the educational materials initially exhibited a more positive response to treatment (week 4), but this difference did not persist at later follow-ups and was associated with significantly higher relapse rates. A strong time-dose relationship was evident between the duration of the initial treatment episode and treatment outcomes at follow-up, but randomized treatment assignment did not influence the duration of initial medication compliance.

Timing: Patients received educational materials in the mail and were periodically assessed by phone after that, for up to 30 weeks of follow-up. The study was conducted from May 1997 to August 1998.

Setting: Three outpatient clinics affiliated with the KPNW healthcare system in Portland, Oregon.

Study design: Randomized, nonblinded intervention study.

Overall risk of study bias: **Moderate to High**

- **Selection bias:** *Low Risk:* 94.8% of the patients asked to be part of the study agreed to take part, and they were randomly assigned to one of the two groups. There is no indication that selection of patients introduced bias in the results of the study. The exclusion criteria of not having access to a touch-tone telephone at home may have introduced bias into sample selection by systematically excluding certain patients (e.g., low socioeconomic status, greater symptom severity, and lower functional ability).
- **Performance bias:** *Low Risk:* There is no evidence of systematic differences in treatment of the study groups. Because the intervention group received the educational materials by mail, it is unlikely that either group received systematically different treatment or cointerventions (e.g., different forms of treatment, varying levels of time or attention).
- **Attrition bias:** *Moderate Risk:* The overall compliance rate for completing the follow-up assessments was 83.2% (614 completed follow-up calls to the IVR system of 738 possible). The compliance rate of patients receiving the RHYTHMS™ materials was slightly higher (85.2%) than the rate for those receiving usual care (81.2%). Those who completed the study may have been more likely to be medication compliant, and this may have introduced bias into the results.
- **Detection bias:** *Low Risk:* Compliance data were confirmed by obtaining prescription fill data from the Kaiser Permanente pharmacy system, and thus outcome assessment was blind to group assignment. Data were obtained using an interactive voice response system on the phone.
- **Reporting bias:** *Low Risk:* There is no evidence of selective outcome reporting.
- **Sponsor-related bias:** *High Risk:* This study was sponsored by Pfizer, which also developed the psychoeducational materials. These materials and sponsorship may have influenced patients' reported compliance with treatment.

Applicability: This study is applicable to the clinical question because patients who received educational materials were compared with those who did not, specifically in the area of compliance with treatment. However, the materials were developed by a pharmaceutical company and may be dissimilar to education provided by a physician or other mental health professional. Also, the study included only patients with depression in a community outpatient setting, which limits applicability of the findings to other diagnoses and settings.

Citation: Myers ED, Branthwaite A: Out-patient compliance with antidepressant medication. *British Journal of Psychiatry* 160:83–86, 1992

Population: The study sample comprised 89 consecutive patients attending a psychiatric outpatient clinic and fulfilling the following criteria: a diagnosis of primary or secondary depression according to the criteria of Feighner et al. (1972), a score of at least 11 on the Ham-D, no clinical evidence of dementia, at least average intelligence as judged by clinical interview, no retardation, and judged to be nonsuicidal.

Intervention: Patients were randomly allocated to each of the three groups, the number allocated to group C being double that allocated to each of the other groups. Group A: One dose of amitriptyline 75 mg or mianserin 30 mg to be taken at night. Group B: Three doses of amitriptyline 25 mg or mianserin 10 mg to be taken during the day. Group C: Either A or B above as chosen by the patient. Those who chose A were designated Group Cn, and those who chose B were designated Group Cd. Mianserin was prescribed rather than amitriptyline if there was considered to be any risk of overdose, albeit without suicide intent.

Comparators: The groups were compared with one another in terms of compliance.

Outcomes: No overall significant difference was found between doctor-prescribed and patient-chosen regimen, or between once-a-day and three-times-a-day dosing. However, compliance was significantly better in those patients who were allowed to choose, when they selected the three-times-a-day regimen. There was a significant decline in compliance for all regimens over the 12 weeks. There was no evidence that better compliance produced a better therapeutic result.

Timing: Twelve-week duration, with assessments at 3, 6, 9, and 12 weeks.

Setting: A psychiatric outpatient clinic in the United Kingdom.

Study design: Randomized clinical trial.

Overall risk of study bias: **Moderate**

- **Selection bias:** *Moderate Risk:* Patients were selected consecutively, rather than randomly, so it is possible that the patients included in the study are not a representative sample. To be included, patients were nonsuicidal, so it is possible that more severe patients were systematically excluded. Patients were also selected for the study on the basis of a diagnosis of depression according to Feighner et al.'s criteria, which may introduce a systematic difference from the diagnosis included in the clinical question.
- **Performance bias:** *Low Risk:* There is no evidence of systematic differences in the treatment of the study groups or of protocol deviation.
- **Attrition bias:** *Moderate Risk:* An intention-to-treat analysis was used, but patients who dropped out are likely to have been less compliant than those who remained in the study.

- **Detection bias:** *Moderate Risk:* Compliance was measured by a series of three questions to the patient and also a pill count. However, because patients are likely to overestimate their compliance, and pill count can be altered by the patient, there is a moderate risk of detection bias.
- **Reporting bias:** *Low Risk:* There is no evidence of selective outcome reporting.
- **Sponsor-related bias:** *Unknown:* There is no information about sponsorship given in the article reporting findings from the study.

Applicability: This study is applicable to the clinical question because it measures the compliance of subjects who had their choice about dosing frequency versus those who did not. However, the choice offered to the subjects was just about dosing frequency, and not about their treatment choices in general, such as which medication they would prefer, or if they would prefer medication at all. This limits the applicability of the overall findings to the clinical question. Also, the study included only patients with a diagnosis of depression receiving treatment in an outpatient setting in the United Kingdom, which may limit applicability to patients with other diagnoses in other treatment settings in the United States.

Citation: Robinson GL, Gilbertson AD, Litwack L: The effects of a psychiatric patient education to medication program on post-discharge compliance. *Psychiatric Quarterly* **58(2):113–118, 1986–1987**

Population: The study subjects consisted of 150 hospitalized patients housed on four acute-care receiving wards and ready for discharge. All of the subjects in the study were voluntary participants who were paid a nominal amount (75¢) for completing the questionnaires required for study inclusion.

Intervention: Patients were randomly assigned to one of three groups: 1) usual care, 2) receiving a 1- to 2-page handout about medications, or 3) receiving the handout plus a verbal review of the information. Subjects were assessed at discharge and at the first follow-up appointment postdischarge.

Comparators: The comparators were patients who received usual care, which included receiving a variable amount of medication-related education but did not include receipt of the handout or specialized verbal reinforcement.

Outcomes: Subjects who received the handout, with or without verbal explanation, showed improvement in understanding of treatment. Subjects who received written information with verbal reinforcement, but not those who received only the handout, were significantly more compliant than the control subjects. There were no significant differences among groups on pretest scores.

Timing: Subjects were assessed at discharge and at their first follow-up appointment at one of four community mental health centers. The mean duration between discharge and the first appointment was 14 days.

Setting: The study was conducted at Fallsview Psychiatric Hospital in Akron, Ohio. Fallsview is a 131-bed state receiving hospital that services a seven-county catchment area. The study was completed in 1986.

Study design: Randomized, single-blind, interventional study.

Overall risk of study bias: **Moderate**

- **Selection bias:** *Low Risk:* patients were randomly assigned to treatment arms, and it appears from the study that all patients at this large state hospital who were ready for discharge were invited to be part of the study. Also, the authors noted that there were no differences between the study groups at pretest.
- **Performance bias:** *Moderate Risk:* The authors noted a potential contamination of the control group with elements of the intervention (i.e., some psychoeducation). However, only the intervention group received the specialized handout and verbal reinforcement.
- **Attrition bias:** *Moderate Risk:* The authors noted that the dropout rate did not appear to differ significantly between groups, but patients who dropped out of the study may have been more likely to be noncompliant with treatment, biasing the results in favor of greater apparent compliance. There was no systematic follow-up with the subjects who dropped out.
- **Detection bias:** *High Risk:* Compliance was measured by a five-question Likert scale ranging from "Never" to "Always" to the question of whether subjects had been compliant with their medications from the hospital. There was no mention of assessing interrater reliability, and despite some information being provided to the clinicians (such as that derived from a patient questionnaire), the compliance ratings are still impressionistic and based on patients' self-report, which may not be reliable.
- **Reporting bias:** *Low Risk:* There is no evidence of selective outcome reporting.
- **Sponsor-related bias:** *Unknown:* There was no mention of sponsorship or funding in the article.

Applicability: This study did answer the clinical question by showing that patients who received more education about risks and benefits of treatment, and specific information about medications, had a higher rate of compliance. The study only concerned hospitalized patients and only evaluated compliance at the first postdischarge visit, and so the range of applicability of the study is somewhat limited. Also, the age of the study (1986) may limit applicability to current treatment.

Citation: Sterling RC, Gottheil E, Glassman SD, et al: Patient treatment choice and compliance: data from a substance abuse treatment program. *American Journal on Addictions/ American Academy of Psychiatrists in Alcoholism and Addictions* **6(2):168–176, 1997**

Population: The study sample comprised 127 patients seeking treatment for cocaine dependence. All of these individuals were being enrolled in treatment at this facility for the first time and had a presentation that met DSM-III-R criteria for cocaine dependence at the time of admission.

Intervention: Subjects received either 12 weeks of weekly individual therapy (IND) or an intensive 3-hour, three-times-per-week treatment program (INT). Half the subjects were given their choice of treatment, and the other half were randomly assigned to one or the other.

Comparators: Patients who had their choice of treatment modality were compared with those who did not have a choice. Because there was no significant pattern of differences between patients receiving IND versus INT, the authors only compared choice and no-choice rather than comparing IND and INT.

Outcomes: Patients who chose IND differed from those who chose INT in only 2 of 41 comparisons: number of previous treatment experiences and ASI Alcohol composite score. Allowing patients to choose their course of treatment did not significantly enhance retention, the proportion of appointments kept, or completion of the 12-week intervention.

Timing: Twelve weeks of treatment, with a 9-month follow-up. The study was conducted in 1997.

Setting: A university-sponsored, publicly funded, community-based, outpatient cocaine treatment program located in a central-city area.

Study design: Randomized, nonblind, interventional study.

Overall risk of study bias: **Moderate**

- **Selection bias:** *Moderate Risk:* Subjects who chose IND versus INT differed on 2 of 41 comparisons: number of previous treatment experiences and ASI Alcohol composite score. The authors noted that the two differences may simply represent chance occurrences. Subjects who did not choose their treatment modality were different on three comparisons—with the differences on all three likely due to chance. Patients were randomly assigned to choice versus no-choice arms, and patients in the no-choice arm were randomly assigned to treatment modality. However, some patients refused to be randomly assigned, mostly because they preferred INT. This may have influenced the results of the study.
- **Performance bias:** *High Risk:* The no-choice condition group was part of a different clinical trial in which participants were randomly assigned to either IND or INT. The choice condition group was treated immediately after this different clinical trial concluded. It is possible that there were systematic differences in the treatment administered to the groups due to experience, attitudinal changes, or other therapist-related factors.
- **Attrition bias:** *Moderate Risk:* The proportion of patients located for the 9-month follow-up interviews did not differ significantly between the choice and no-choice groups (60% and 76%, respectively), but an administrative lapse (per the authors) led to follow-up not being sought for the final 11 cases in the randomly assigned (no-choice) condition. This may have affected results, but the effects of this are unclear.
- **Detection bias:** *High Risk:* Several of the outcome measures were obtained through patient interview, such as addiction severity, AIDS risk behavior, days of cocaine use, and so forth. Patients may underreport (or overreport) these data, leading to detection bias.
- **Reporting bias:** *Low Risk:* There is no evidence of selective outcome reporting.
- **Sponsor-related bias:** *Low Risk:* This research was supported in part by a grant from the National Institute on Drug Abuse (NIDA) and performed under the auspices of the Commonwealth Office of Drug and Alcohol Programs (ODAP) and the Philadelphia Department of Public Health, Coordinating Office for Drug and Alcohol Abuse Program (CODAAP).

Applicability: The study is applicable to the clinical question in that it assessed the effect of offering treatment choice on retention in treatment, which is a form of adherence. The study only concerns patients seeking substance abuse treatment, so the scope of the study is fairly narrow and does not apply to all psychiatric patients.

Citation: Vandereycken W, Vansteenkiste M: Let eating disorder patients decide: providing choice may reduce early drop-out from inpatient treatment. *European Eating Disorders Review* **17(3):177–183, 2009**

Population: The study population consisted of inpatients on a specialized female-only eating disorders unit. There were 87 patients in the intervention arm and 87 control patients.

Intervention: Eighty-seven patients who underwent a new admission strategy that emphasized patent choice were compared with 87 controls who were admitted prior to implementation of the new strategy. The old strategy involved patients starting in an observation group for 1–2 weeks. Staff made decisions about treatment and attempted to motivate the patient to accept the treatment provision. The new strategy involved all patients starting with an admission interview, followed by a tour of the unit and an explanation of the program. The patient came for a 5-day introductory week and then made a decision about whether to continue with treatment. No attempts were made to change the patient's mind if she opted to refuse further care.

Comparators: Eighty-seven prior admissions before the new admission strategy was adopted in 2001.

Outcomes: The results indicate that the provision of choice at the beginning of treatment significantly reduced the number of dropouts during the first weeks of inpatient treatment. No differences were found between strategies on later dropping out and weight change (in anorexia nervosa patients) during inpatient treatment.

Timing: Data were gathered from 2002 to 2004. The admission strategy involved a 5-day introductory period prior to entering treatment.

Setting: A 35-bed specialized female-only inpatient treatment unit for eating disorder patients.

Study design: Quasi-experimental design that compared patients before and after a new treatment strategy was introduced. The study is a retrospective chart review.

Overall risk of study bias: **Moderate**

- **Selection bias:** *Low Risk:* There is no discussion of consenting patients to the study, because the study was a chart review only. There were no exclusion criteria per se, and it seems as if the authors chose all patients (in the intervention arm) during a particular period and then matched them with controls.
- **Performance bias:** *High Risk:* There is no evidence of systematic differences in the treatment of the groups before and after implementation of the new strategy. However, unreported factors, such as staff enthusiasm for the new approach, may have been present, and the study design would not eliminate such confounding effects.
- **Attrition bias:** *Low Risk:* Not applicable, because patients were not followed over time; rather, this was a retrospective chart review.
- **Detection bias:** *Low Risk:* The two outcome variables were dropout rates and weight change. It does not appear that either variable would have been subject to detection bias.
- **Reporting bias:** *Low Risk:* There is no evidence of selective outcome reporting.
- **Sponsor-related bias:** *Unknown:* There was no mention of sponsorship in the article.

Applicability: The study is applicable to the clinical question because it focuses on dropout rates (adherence) in patients who were given more versus less choice in their treatment. However, this study is concerned with a narrow range of patients (e.g., all female, all with eating disorders, all inpatient), which limits the applicability of its findings to psychiatric patients in general. Also, the study was conducted in Belgium, and so the effects of additional choice on this population may be different for a U.S. patient population.

Citation: Vreeland B, Minsky S, Yanos PT, et al.: Efficacy of the team solutions program for educating patients about illness management and treatment. *Psychiatric Services* 57(6):822–828, 2006

Population: The study population comprised 71 outpatients with schizophrenia or schizoaffective disorder from day-treatment settings.

Intervention: Patients were randomly assigned either to a 24-week comprehensive, modularized, psychoeducational intervention focused on illness management called Team Solutions or to standard care. The intervention involved attending a Team Solutions meeting twice a day, two days a week, for 24 weeks. Each meeting lasted 1 hour.

Comparators: Patients randomly assigned to standard care.

Outcomes: Attendance at the meetings varied from 20% to 94%, with a mean of 73%. Significant improvement was observed in knowledge about schizophrenia and client satisfaction in the intervention group. No changes were observed in symptoms, treatment adherence, or global functioning.

Timing: Twenty-four-week intervention. Data were collected from September 2002 to September 2003.

Setting: The University of Medicine and Dentistry of New Jersey–University Behavioral HealthCare (a statewide mental health care delivery system at the university).

Study design: Single-blind, randomized controlled trial.

Overall risk of study bias: **Moderate**

- **Selection bias:** *Moderate Risk:* Exclusion criteria included dementia, mental retardation or intellectual impairment, suicidality, and exposure to more than one Team Solutions workbook. All subjects had to have attended the partial hospitalization program for at least 2 days. Because subjects had to provide consent and be willing to participate in a rigorous 24-week intervention, the participants may not have represented all patients with schizophrenia or schizoaffective disorder.
- **Performance bias:** *Moderate Risk:* This study was not blinded to the subjects, and so responses may have been affected by knowledge of which treatment arm the subject was in (e.g., knowing that a subject participated in the psychoeducational group, that subject may report that he or she has more knowledge about schizophrenia). The authors noted that the day-treatment programs from which participants were recruited included some psychoeducational services, which may have introduced bias from contamination of the control group with exposure to the intervention.
- **Attrition bias:** *Moderate Risk:* Data were analyzed with a linear random coefficient regression model for repeated measures, which is "in line with an intention-to-treat analysis." However, there was no discussion of number of dropouts from the study, and it would seem that there would be dropouts because of the length of the intervention (24 weeks). Those who dropped out may have been less likely to score well on tests assessing knowledge of schizophrenia.
- **Detection bias:** *Low Risk:* The authors reported that the questionnaires used in the study have good reliability overall.
- **Reporting bias:** *Low Risk:* There is no evidence of selective outcome reporting.
- **Sponsor-related bias:** *Moderate Risk:* The project was funded in part by Eli Lilly and Company, which could have introduced bias into the study design or results.

Applicability: This study has overall applicability to the clinical question, although it only focused on patients with a particular set of diagnoses.

Grading of Supporting Body of Research Evidence

Risk of bias: Studies varied in risk of bias from low to high. However, overall, most studies had moderate risk. The body of research evidence is made up of many randomized controlled trials and several observational studies. However, pooling of data for each outcome is difficult because of study heterogeneity.

Consistency: **Inconsistent:** The interventions in the studies varied widely, as did the outcome measures and the results of the studies. Some studies found that involvement of the patient in treatment decision making improved adherence to treatment, but others did not find that. Some found that patient choice improved clinical outcomes, whereas others did not. Generally, when patients were educated about their illness or treatment, measurements showed that their knowledge increased. Typically, patient satisfaction improved when there was more contact with the treatment teams but this was not necessarily the case when information was conveyed by printed materials only.

Directness: **Indirect:** Many studies directly measured adherence and patient satisfaction after an intervention in which patients were educated or included in a decision-making intervention. However, because the interventions were highly varied, and the populations studied were often very different and covered specific diagnoses, the studies overall are indirect when it comes to answering the clinical question.

Precision: **Imprecise:** The studies have variable outcomes, and the outcome measures evaluated (e.g., treatment adherence, attitudes toward treatment, satisfaction with treatment, therapeutic alliance) are subjective, qualitative, and difficult to measure.

Dose-response relationship: **Not applicable:** It did appear overall that interventions which involved the patient in treatment improved adherence and satisfaction. However, because the interventions were highly varied, and because none of the studies evaluated various "doses" or quantities of interventions, this could not be evaluated.

Magnitude of effect: **Weak:** Generally, it appears that there is only a modest effect on adherence and therapeutic alliance when decision-making interventions are implemented. This may be because "standard care," which was the comparator to these interventions, is not at all uniform. Standard care generally also involves treatment discussions and involvement of the patient in care decisions.

Confounding factors (including likely direction of effect):   Because researchers, study participants, and subjects all knew they were involved in studies assessing patient adherence and alliance based on an intervention of some kind versus standard care, many sources of bias and confounding factors may have influenced results. For example, clinicians performing "standard care" in these studies may have been more diligent about involving patients in decision making because these patients were being monitored. It is not always clear whether the same clinicians were providing the intervention and the standard care conditions, which could also have led to shifts in the actual delivered intervention or the way in which standard care was done.

Publication bias: **Not able to be assessed.**

Applicability: Some studies were not very applicable to the clinical question either because the outcome measures were not exactly related to the clinical question or because the patient population and treatment setting being studied were too narrow. However, several studies did appear to answer the question.

Overall strength of research evidence: **Low.**

Differences of Opinion in Rating the Strength of Recommendations

None.

Expert Opinion Survey Results

To what extent do you agree that the therapeutic alliance and treatment adherence are improved by explaining the following to patients who have the capacity for decision making?

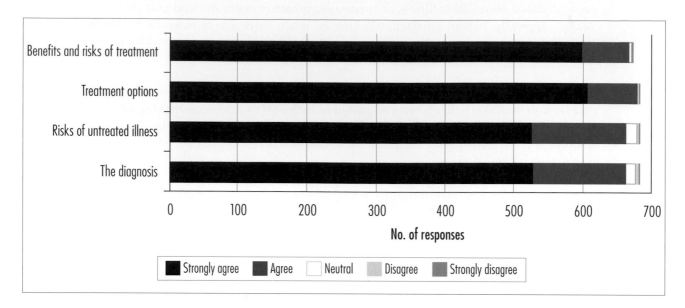

Percentage of experts who "strongly agreed" or "agreed" that therapeutic alliance and treatment adherence are improved by explaining the following to patients who have the capacity for decision making:

Benefits and risks of treatment	99.3%
Treatment options	99.4%
Risks of untreated illness	97.1%
The diagnosis	96.9%

Do you typically (i.e., almost always) explain these items to your patients who have the capacity for decision making?

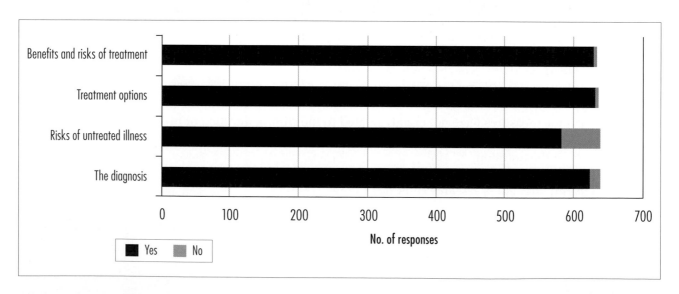

For patients with the capacity for decision making, to what extent do you agree that the therapeutic alliance and treatment adherence are improved by asking about treatment-related preferences?

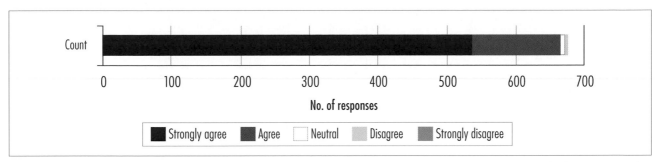

Percentage of experts who "strongly agreed" or "agreed" that for patients with the capacity for decision making, the therapeutic alliance and treatment adherence are improved by asking about treatment-related preferences: 98.4%.

Do you typically (i.e., almost always) ask your patients who have the capacity for decision making about their preferences regarding available treatment options?

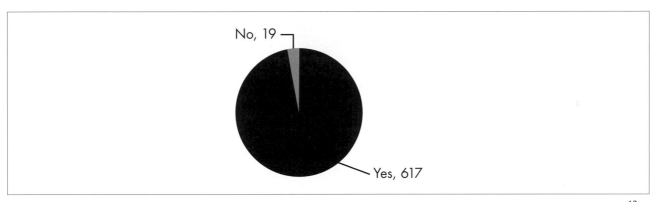

To what extent do you agree that the following are improved by "shared decision making"?[12]

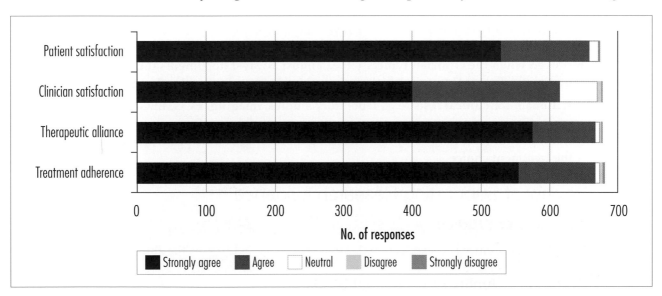

---

[12] "Shared decision making" is defined as collaboration between clinicians and patients about decisions pertinent to treatment, when the patient has capacity for decision making.

Percentage of experts who "strongly agreed" or "agreed" that the following are improved by "shared decision making":

Patient satisfaction	97.5%
Clinician satisfaction	90.9%
Therapeutic alliance	98.4%
Treatment adherence	97.9%

Do you typically (i.e., almost always) collaborate with your patients in decision making regarding treatment?

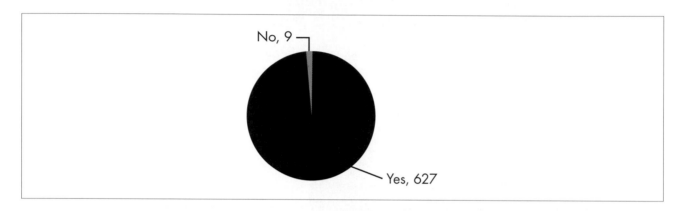

GUIDELINE IX. Documentation of the Psychiatric Evaluation

Clinical Question

Development of this guideline was premised on the following clinical question:

For patients who present with a psychiatric symptom, sign, or syndrome in any setting, is an individual clinician's decision making about a patient's psychiatric diagnosis and treatment plan improved when the clinician typically (i.e., almost always) documents the following in the patient's medical record? Is coordination of psychiatric treatment with other clinicians improved?

- **Rationale for clinical tests (e.g., laboratory studies, imaging, ECG, EEG) as part of the initial evaluation**
- **Rationale for treatment selection, including discussion of the specific factors that influenced the treatment choice**

Review of Supporting Research Evidence

Overview of Studies

There is no supporting research evidence that specifically addresses the above clinical question.

Grading of Quality of Individual Studies

Not applicable.

Grading of Supporting Body of Research Evidence

Not applicable.

Differences of Opinion in Rating the Strength of Recommendations

One member of the work group was uncertain that potential benefits of documenting the rationale for treatment selection clearly outweigh harms. This difference of opinion is considered minor.

Expert Opinion Survey Results

To what extent do you agree that an individual clinician's decision making about a patient's psychiatric diagnosis and treatment plan is improved when the clinician typically (i.e., almost always) documents the following in the patient's medical record?

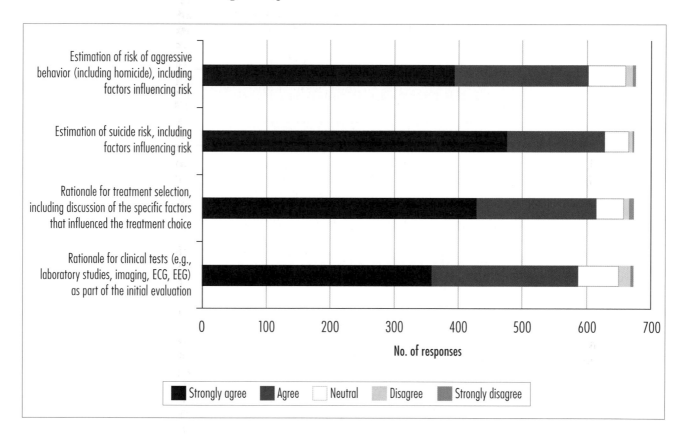

Percentage of experts who "strongly agreed" or "agreed" that an individual clinician's decision making about a patient's psychiatric diagnosis and treatment plan is improved when the clinician typically (i.e., almost always) documents the following in the patient's medical record:

Estimation of risk of aggressive behavior (including homicide), including factors influencing risk	89.3%
Estimation of suicide risk, including factors influencing risk	93.2%
Rationale for treatment selection, including discussion of the specific factors that influenced the treatment choice	91.4%
Rationale for clinical tests (e.g., laboratory studies, imaging, ECG, EEG) as part of the initial evaluation	86.9%

To what extent do you agree that coordination of psychiatric treatment with other clinicians is improved when these same items are typically (i.e., almost always) documented?

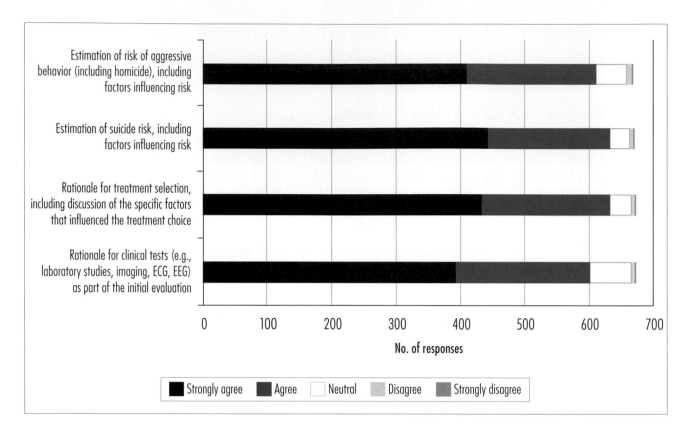

Percentage of experts who "strongly agreed" or "agreed" that coordination of psychiatric treatment with other clinicians is improved when these same items are typically (i.e., almost always) documented:

Estimation of risk of aggressive behavior (including homicide), including factors influencing risk	91.3%
Estimation of suicide risk, including factors influencing risk	94.5%
Rationale for treatment selection, including discussion of the specific factors that influenced the treatment choice	93.8%
Rationale for clinical tests (e.g., laboratory studies, imaging, ECG, EEG) as part of the initial evaluation	89.5%

Do you typically (i.e., almost always) document these items in the medical record of your patients?

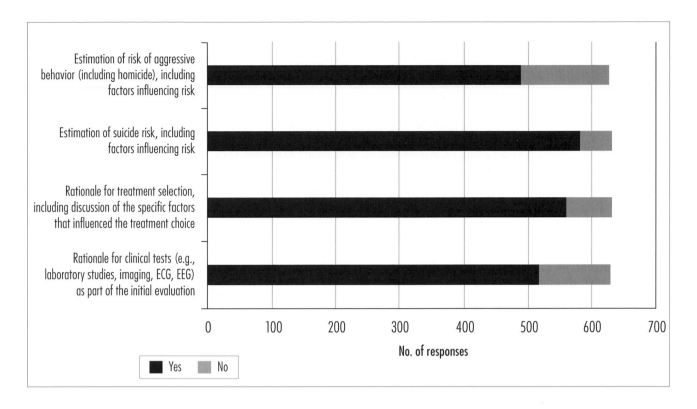

Quality Measurement Considerations
GUIDELINE I. Review of Psychiatric Symptoms, Trauma History, and Psychiatric Treatment History

This guideline recommends that the initial psychiatric evaluation include a review of the patient's mood, level of anxiety, thought content and process, and perception and cognition (statement 1); trauma history (statement 2); and psychiatric treatment history (statement 3). As described under "Expert Opinion Survey Results," expert psychiatrists typically practice in very high accordance with these recommendations. The typical practices of other psychiatrists are unknown, but these assessments are understood to be standard components of an initial psychiatric evaluation. As a result, quality improvement activities including performance measures that are derived from this guideline may not yield substantial improvements in quality of care that would justify increased clinician burden (e.g., documentation burden).

There are important practical barriers to deriving quality measures from statement 3 (assessment of psychiatric treatment history). For example, to assess a clinician's performance of a clinical process, a measure must clearly define the applicable patient group (i.e., the denominator) and the process that is measured (i.e., the numerator). Unlike an outcome measure, a process measure should not depend on the patient's response or report. Furthermore, the clinician's performance of the process must be readily ascertained from chart review or administrative data. For these reasons, it would be impractical to measure the process of assessing a patient's psychiatric treatment history. As described under "Implementation," patients may not know or be able to recall their previous diagnoses or past treatment trials, nor their level of adherence or response to past treatments. Furthermore, information in medical records may be lacking or incomplete.

Although there may be little to gain in deriving measures from statements 1 and 2, practical barriers are less challenging and relate mainly to a lack of standardization in how findings about psychiatric signs, symptoms, and trauma history are documented. As described under "Implementation," there are many possible clinical approaches and questions that might be used to conduct these assessments, and oversimplification is a possible unintended consequence of measurement. One approach that may minimize this risk could be to measure for the presence or absence of text only in relevant fields of the medical record (e.g., fields for mood, level of anxiety, thought content and process, perception and cognition). This approach would allow for maximum flexibility in how clinicians document findings of their assessments. Alternatively, a measure could consider the presence or absence of scoring from a relevant measurement tool. As described under "Implementation," the DSM-5 Level 1 Cross-Cutting Symptom Measure (American Psychiatric Association 2013b) addresses domains that overlap with the assessment items recommended in statement 1. Exceptions to the denominator of performance measures derived from this guideline might include patients who are unable to participate in the evaluation due to current mental status. Other exceptions may also be appropriate.

Ideally, measures that aim to improve the assessment of specific health conditions should be paired with measures that aim to improve the use of effective treatments whenever the condition is identified. Recommendations about follow-up are out of scope for this guideline. However, there may be opportunities to pair assessment measures derived from this guideline with follow-up measures derived from other guidelines.

GUIDELINE II. Substance Use Assessment

This guideline recommends that the initial psychiatric evaluation of a patient include assessment of the patient's use of tobacco, alcohol, or other substances (e.g., marijuana, cocaine, heroin, hallucinogens) and any misuse of prescribed or over-the-counter (OTC) medications or supplements. As described under "Expert Opinion Survey Results," expert psychiatrists typically practice in accordance with this recommendation. Among psychiatrists practicing in ambulatory settings, rates of tobacco use screening have been declining and rates of treatment for smoking cessation are low (Rogers and Sherman 2014). The typical practices of other psychiatrists and mental health professionals are unknown, but these professionals may conduct substance use assessments to varying degrees and through various methods in initial evaluations. This variability could indicate a need to strengthen clinician knowledge, improve training, and increase the time and attention that clinicians give to substance use assessment. Furthermore, there may be opportunities to improve quality in these areas for patients across healthcare settings, not just mental health.

As described under "Implementation," the clinical approach and specific questions used to assess substance use may vary. For many patients, substance use may be adequately assessed with a series of straightforward questions or through the use of a standardized questionnaire or self-report scales. For other patients, an individualized approach may be needed. Quality improvement activities derived from this guideline, including performance measures, should not oversimplify the process of assessing substance use. For example, quality improvement activities may aim to ensure that assessment has occurred and is documented in a patient's record but should avoid specifying use of a specific method of assessment (e.g., a specific scale). This approach is consistent with two existing measures endorsed by the National Quality Forum (NQF): NQF Measure 028, "Preventive Care & Screening: Tobacco Use: Screening & Cessation Intervention," assesses the percentage of adult patients who are screened every 2 years for tobacco use and who receive cessation counseling intervention if identified as a tobacco user (http://www.qualityforum.org/QPS/0028). NQF Measure 110, "Bipolar Disorder and Major Depression: Appraisal for Alcohol or Chemical Substance Use," assesses the percentage of patients with depression or bipolar disorder with evidence of an initial assessment that includes an appraisal for alcohol or chemical substance use (http://www.qualityforum.org/QPS/0110).

Although both of these NQF-endorsed measures are consistent with this guideline, a more comprehensive measure could also be derived that assesses the percentage of patients seen in an initial psychiatric evaluation who are screened for the use of tobacco, alcohol, or other substances as well as for the misuse of prescribed or OTC medications. Such a measure could be implemented by measuring for the presence or absence of text in fields labeled "tobacco use," "alcohol use," "other substance use," and "misuse of prescribed or over-the-counter medications." This approach would allow for maximum flexibility in how clinicians document findings of their assessments. Alternatively, a measure could consider the presence or absence of scoring from a relevant measurement tool. Exceptions to the denominator of the measure might include individuals who have already been diagnosed with a substance use disorder or patients who are unable to participate in the evaluation because of their current mental status. Other exceptions might also be appropriate.

Ideally, measures that aim to improve the assessment of specific health conditions should be paired with measures that aim to improve the use of effective treatments whenever the condition is identified. Recommendations about follow-up for patients who have a substance use disorder are out of scope for this guideline. However, there may be opportunities to pair assessment measures derived from this guideline with follow-up measures derived from other guidelines.

GUIDELINE III. Assessment of Suicide Risk

This guideline recommends that the initial psychiatric evaluation of a patient include assessment of key factors associated with increased suicide risk. It also recommends documentation of an overall estimation of suicide risk, which is a matter of clinical judgment that is informed by all data collected about an individual patient during the evaluation. As described under "Expert Opinion Survey Results," expert psychiatrists typically practice in accordance with these recommendations. The typical practices of other psychiatrists and mental health professionals are unknown, but these professionals may assess suicide risk to varying degrees and through various methods. Variability also seems common in how suicide risk is documented—for example, some medical records provide a clear description of the clinician's judgment about a patient's level of risk, whereas other records only indicate "+SI" or "–SI." This variability could indicate a need to strengthen clinician knowledge about suicide risk factors, improve training about how to conduct a suicide risk assessment, and increase the time and attention that clinicians give to suicide risk assessment, including making an overall estimation of risk.

Quality improvement activities derived from this guideline, including performance measures, must not oversimplify the process of assessing suicide risk factors and formulating an estimation about overall risk. This guideline is not intended to represent a comprehensive set of questions relating to suicide risk assessment, nor is it intended to suggest that assessment can or should be reduced to a series of yes or no questions. As described under "Implementation," there are a variety of ways clinicians may obtain recommended information about risk factors. In addition, assessment may be compromised by practical barriers such as a patient's inability to communicate. Many risk factors are difficult to define and may even be impossible to quantify or assess in a standardized way. Clinical judgment must determine which factors merit emphasis in the assessment of an individual patient, and clinical judgment is necessary to synthesize information and observations about the individual patient into an estimation of overall risk.

For these reasons, it would be inappropriate for quality improvement purposes to implement this guideline as a requirement that all of the recommended risk factors and an overall estimation of risk must be documented for all patients who receive an initial psychiatric evaluation. Furthermore, as described under "Implementation," no standardized scale for assessing risk has been shown to have clinically useful specificity, sensitivity, or predictive value. As a result, many clinicians appropriately use free text prose to describe a patient's suicide risk. Reviewing these free text records for measurement purposes would be impractical.

An approach that considers the above issues could be to measure for the presence or absence of a body of text under a field labeled "suicide risk estimation" in the patient's medical record, without addressing the content of the text. This approach would require that an estimation of suicide risk be formulated into words and documented, but it would not burden the clinician to assess and record risk in a specific, inflexible way. As documentation of suicide risk becomes increasingly standardized and natural language processing becomes increasingly sophisticated, a measure on the specific content of the analysis could be considered.

A liability of this approach is that it would have limited utility to address variability in how clinicians assess and document risk. This approach could also have unintended consequences: As described under "Potential Benefits and Harms," when the amount of time available for an evaluation is constrained, time used to focus on assessment of suicide risk could reduce time available to address other issues of importance to the patient. This possible unintended consequence could be addressed in testing of a fully specified measure.

An alternative approach could be to measure for clinician documentation of risk factors that are typically recorded in an electronic medical record in a standardized way (e.g., presence or absence of current suicidal ideas, prior hospitalization, substance use, and psychosocial stressors). Advantages of this approach include practicality and feasibility and the potential to address specific knowledge deficits (e.g., knowledge that prior hospitalization increases suicide risk). Clinicians might also find a measure that takes this approach to be less burdensome. The main disadvantage of this approach is that it could lead clinicians to focus on the measured factors rather than other, equally important or potentially more important factors that are not measured.

In clinical practice, because of the overlap in risk factors for suicide and aggression, risk is often assessed simultaneously, and an estimation of risk for either suicide or aggression or both is documented in the same paragraph or field in the medical record. As a result, a measure on suicide risk assessment might be paired, combined, or harmonized with a measure on aggression risk assessment.

Ideally, measures that aim to improve the assessment of specific health conditions should be paired with measures that aim to improve the use of effective treatments whenever the condition is identified. Recommendations about follow-up, and derived measures, are out of scope for this guideline. However, there may be opportunities to pair assessment measures derived from this guideline with follow-up measures derived from other guidelines.

GUIDELINE IV. Assessment of Risk for Aggressive Behaviors

This guideline recommends assessment of key factors associated with increased risk for aggressive behaviors in patients who are receiving an initial psychiatric evaluation. It suggests documentation of an overall estimation of risk, which is a matter of clinical judgment that is informed by all data collected about an individual patient during the evaluation.

As described under "Expert Opinion Survey: Results," expert psychiatrists typically practice in accordance with these recommendations. The typical practices of other psychiatrists and mental health professionals are unknown. Anecdotal observations suggest that they may assess risk to varying degrees and through various methods. Variability in how risk is documented also seems common. This variability could indicate a need to strengthen clinician knowledge about risk factors, improve training about how to conduct a risk assessment, and increase the time and attention that clinicians give to assessment, including making an overall estimation of risk.

Quality improvement activities derived from this guideline, including performance measures, must not oversimplify the process of assessing risk factors for aggressive behaviors and formulating an estimation about overall risk. This guideline is not intended to represent a comprehensive set of questions relating to risk assessment, nor is this intended to suggest that assessment can or should be reduced to a series of yes or no questions. As described under "Implementation," there are a variety of ways clinicians may obtain recommended information about risk factors. In addition, assessment may be compromised by practical barriers such as a patient's inability to communicate. Many risk factors are difficult to define and may even be impossible to quantify or assess in a standardized way. Clinical judgment must determine which factors merit emphasis in the assessment of an individual patient, and clinical judgment is necessary to synthesize information and observations about the individual patient into an estimation of overall risk.

For these reasons, it would be inappropriate for quality improvement purposes to implement this guideline as a requirement that all of the recommended risk factors and an overall estimation of risk must be documented for all patients who receive an initial psychiatric evaluation. Furthermore, as described under "Implementation," no standardized instrument for assessing risk has been shown to have predictive validity. As a result, many clinicians appropriately use free text prose to describe a patient's risk. Reviewing these free text records for measurement purposes would be impractical.

An approach that considers the issues discussed above could be to measure for the presence or absence of a body of text under a field labeled "Estimation of Risk for Aggressive Behaviors" in the patient's medical record, without addressing the content of the text. This approach would require that an estimation of risk be formulated into words and documented, but it would not burden the clinician to assess and record risk in a specific, inflexible way. As documentation of risk becomes increasingly standardized and natural language processing becomes increasingly sophisticated, a measure on the specific content of the analysis could be considered.

A liability of this approach is that it would have limited utility to address variability in how clinicians assess and document risk. This approach could also have unintended consequences: As described under "Potential Benefits and Harms," when the amount of time available for an evaluation is constrained, time used to focus on assessment of risk of aggressive behaviors could reduce time available to address other issues of importance to the patient. This possible unintended consequence could be addressed in testing of a fully specified measure.

An alternative approach could be to measure for clinician documentation of risk factors that are typically recorded in an electronic medical record in a standardized way (e.g., prior emergency visits or psychiatric hospitalization, substance use, psychosocial stressors). Advantages of this approach include practicality and feasibility and the potential to address specific knowledge deficits (e.g., knowledge that prior hospitalization increases risk). Clinicians might also find a measure that takes this approach to be less burdensome. The main disadvantage of this approach is that it could lead clinicians to focus on the measured factors rather than other, equally important or potentially more important factors that are not measured. In addition, this approach may not encourage clinicians to formulate an overall estimation of risk of aggressive behaviors, as information on these independent risk factors may be collected for other reasons, such as to assess suicide risk or substance use.

In clinical practice, because of the overlap in risk factors for suicide and aggression, risk is often assessed simultaneously, and an estimation of risk for either suicide or aggression or both is documented in the same paragraph or field in the medical record. As a result, a measure on aggression risk assessment might be paired, combined, or harmonized with a measure on suicide risk assessment.

Ideally, measures that aim to improve the assessment of specific health conditions should be paired with measures that aim to improve the use of effective treatments whenever the condition is identified. Recommendations about follow-up, and derived measures, are out of scope for this guideline. However, there may be opportunities to pair measures derived from this guideline with follow-up measures derived from other guidelines.

GUIDELINE V. Assessment of Cultural Factors

This guideline recommends that an initial psychiatric evaluation include assessment of a patient's language needs for an interpreter (statement 1) and cultural factors related to the patient's social environment (statement 2). Assessment of the patient's personal/cultural beliefs and cultural explanations of psychiatric illness is suggested (statement 3). As described under "Expert Opinion Survey Results," expert psychiatrists typically practice in accordance with these recommendations. The typical practices of other psychiatrists and mental health professionals are unknown. Anecdotal observations suggest that they may conduct language and cultural assessments to varying degrees and through various methods. This variability could indicate a need to strengthen clinician knowledge, improve training, and increase the time and attention that clinicians give to language and cultural assessment. Furthermore, there may be opportunities to improve quality in these areas for patients across healthcare settings, not just mental health.

As described under "Implementation," for many patients, language needs can be easily determined. For others, assessment may include establishing both the need for an interpreter and the appropriateness of different interpreter options. Three aspects of language assessment are therefore suggested as the possible focus of quality measures derived from statement 1: assessing the patient's primary language, asking about interpreter preference, and using an interpreter when appropriate. With respect to assessing primary language, a measure endorsed by the National Quality Forum (NQF) is available that assesses the percent of patient visits and admissions where preferred spoken language for health care is screened and recorded (NQF Measure 1824, "Language Services: The Percent of Patient Visits and Admissions Where Preferred Spoken Language for Health Care Is Screened and Recorded"; www.qualitymeasures.ahrq.gov/content.aspx?id=27294). A similar measure might assess the percentage of patient visits and admissions where interpreter preference is screened and recorded. With respect to using an interpreter, an NQF-endorsed measure is available that assesses the percentage of limited English-proficient patients receiving both initial assessment and discharge instructions supported by assessed and trained interpreters or from bilingual providers and bilingual workers/employees assessed for language proficiency (NQF Measure 1821, "Language Services: The Percent of Limited English-Proficient (LEP) Patients Receiving Both Initial Assessment and Discharge Instructions Supported by Assessed and Trained Interpreters or From Bilingual Providers and Bilingual Workers/Employees Assessed for Language Proficiency"; http://www.qualitymeasures.ahrq.gov/content.aspx?id=27296).

Unlike language needs, personal and cultural factors, beliefs, and explanations of illness are highly variable and not well defined; there are a variety of appropriate ways clinicians may obtain recommended information; and there are a number of potential barriers to conducting the assessment. It would therefore be difficult to derive meaningful performance measures from either statement 2 or statement 3, and it would be inappropriate to hold clinicians accountable to such measures. However, quality of care might be improved through other activities derived from these statements, such as educational activities.

GUIDELINE VI. Assessment of Medical Health

This guideline recommends that the initial psychiatric evaluation of a patient include assessment of whether or not the patient has an ongoing relationship with a primary health care professional (statement 1). Also recommended is assessment of specific aspects of the patient's medical health (statement 2) as well as all medications the patient is currently taking or was recently taking and the side effects of those medications (statement 3). Although many health care professionals may participate in the evaluation of patients with mental illness, including psychologists, social workers, and nurse practitioners, statements 2 and 3 have greatest applicability to medically trained clinicians. As described under "Expert Opinion Survey Results," expert psychiatrists frequently practice in accordance with the recommendations of this guideline. The typical practices of other psychiatrists are unknown, but anecdotal observations suggest possible variability. This variability could indicate a need to strengthen knowledge, improve training, and increase the time and attention that psychiatrists give to the assessment of patients' medical status in initial evaluations. Furthermore, there may be opportunities to improve quality in these areas for patients seen by physicians in other fields of medicine.

With respect to statement 1, assessment is straightforward, and the information collected is typically recorded in medical records in a standardized way (i.e., the name of the primary health care professional or primary care clinic). One approach to measurement could be to evaluate the number of patients who receive a psychiatric evaluation for whom the name of the patient's primary care health professional or primary care clinic is documented. Exceptions could include patients who report that they do not see a primary care professional, who cannot recall the name of the clinician or clinic, or who are unable to report this information because of current psychiatric symptoms. Because these exceptions occur frequently in many settings, the approach to implementation might involve measuring for the presence or absence of any text in a field labeled "primary health care professional" rather than for the presence or absence of a specific name. A paired measure could be developed to encourage, whenever "none" or "unknown" is documented, follow-up with such patients to establish a relationship with a primary health care professional. Statement 1 could also inform a more generic measure intended to promote coordination of care across all fields of medicine.

As described under "Implementation," there are many possible clinical approaches and questions that might be used to assess the aspects of medical health described in statement 2. For some patients, particularly those with no serious medical conditions, the recommended items could be assessed through a series of simple questions or through the use of a standardized form. For other patients, especially those with serious medical illnesses co-occurring with a psychiatric condition, a more thorough and individualized approach could be needed. For this reason, quality improvement activities derived from statement 2, including performance measures, should not oversimplify the process of assessment. One approach, for example, might be to measure whether or not the recommended aspects of the patient's medical health are assessed but not how they are assessed or how findings are documented. There are important practical challenges with this approach. For example, implementation would minimally require that a clinician's medical record capture yes or no as to whether each item was considered during the evaluation. Not all medical records may do this, and even if they do, information may not be captured in an easily retrievable format. Furthermore, findings may not typically be documented unless abnormal, and some abnormalities may not be documented if they are not important for the patient's diagnosis and treatment (e.g., tonsillectomy, nearsightedness). Finally, an important unintended consequence of this approach to measurement, particularly if implemented as a measure of the presence or absence of text within nine separate fields of the medical record, could be that clinicians use time and resources to document findings that are not relevant to a patient's care. Furthermore, such documentation would be distracting to readers of notes and impede clinical thought processes and decision making.

There are also important practical challenges with respect to statement 3 that could make this recommendation unsuitable for implementation as a performance measure. The presence of a list of medications in the patient's medical record is in itself a poor indicator of how thoroughly a clinician has inquired about all medications, including nonprescribed medications, and how diligently the clinician has considered side effects and drug interactions of those medications in relation to differential diagnosis and treatment planning. However, it is worth noting that the recommendation is consistent with two measures endorsed by the NQF: Measure 0097, "Medication Reconciliation" (http://www.qualityforum.org/QPS/0097), and Measure 0553, "Care for Older Adults—Medication Review" (http://www.qualityforum.org/QPS/0553). NQF Measure 0097 considers the percentage of patients 18 years and older discharged from any inpatient facility and seen within 30 days of discharge in the office by the physician, prescribing practitioner, registered nurse, or clinical pharmacist who had a documented reconciliation of the discharge medications with the current medication list in the outpatient medical record. NQF Measure 0553 considers the percentage of adults age 66 years and older who had a medication review in the past year and for whom the medical record includes a list of medications.

Statements 4 and 5 are not appropriate for quality measurement because the balance of benefits and harms of the suggested assessments is uncertain.

Ideally, measures that aim to improve the assessment of specific health conditions should be paired with measures that aim to improve the use of effective treatments whenever the condition is identified. Recommendations about follow-up, and derived measures, are out of scope for this guideline. However, there may be opportunities to pair assessment measures derived from this guideline with follow-up measures derived from other guidelines.

GUIDELINE VII. Quantitative Assessment

This guideline is not appropriate for quality measurement because the balance of benefits and harms of the suggested assessments is uncertain.

GUIDELINE VIII. Involvement of the Patient in Treatment Decision Making

This guideline recommends that the initial psychiatric evaluation of a patient who is seen and who has capacity for decision making include an explanation of the following: the differential diagnosis, risks of untreated illness, treatment options, and benefits and risks of treatment (statement 1). Also recommended are that the evaluation include asking the patient about treatment-related preferences (statement 2) and that the clinician collaborate with the patient about decisions pertinent to treatment (statement 3).

As described under "Expert Opinion Survey: Results," expert psychiatrists typically practice in very high accordance with this guideline. The typical practices of other psychiatrists are unknown, but similar high accordance might be expected on the basis that shared decision making is commonly understood to be a principle of ethical practice, as described under "Rationale." As a result, quality improvement activities including performance measures that are derived from this guideline may not yield substantial improvements in quality of care that would justify increased clinician burden (e.g., documentation burden).

Measures on the use of shared decision making have been endorsed by the NQF. For example, NQF Measure 0310, "Back Pain: Shared Decision Making" (http://www.qualityforum.org/QPS/0310) considers if the medical record of a patient with back pain includes documentation that a discussion occurred between the physician and the patient, prior to surgery, of the following: 1) treatment choices, including alternatives to surgery; 2) risks and benefits; and 3) evidence of effectiveness.

Quality measures such as NQF Measure 0310 that aim to promote shared decision making are consistent with the stated goal of this guideline but have serious practical limitations. As described under "Implementation," the use of shared decision-making approaches within an initial psychiatric evaluation depends on the individual patient and the clinical context. A priori, the capacity of the patient to collaborate must be evaluated by the clinician. This judgment is by nature a nuanced process and is subject to change over time (e.g., as psychiatric symptoms emerge or subside). Even when a patient is judged to have the capacity to collaborate, the level of collaboration that is possible may vary (e.g., depending on the patient's level of insight about his or her psychiatric illness and need for treatment). Collaboration may also vary according to the patient's preferences. For these reasons, shared decision making is an inherently complex and individualized process, and it would be impractical to document in a standardized way when and to what degree shared decision-making occurs. A checkbox approach, for example, would be undesirable for the purposes of performance measurement because of possible clinician bias and overreporting of measure adherence. Patient-reported data might augment clinician-reported data but could also introduce bias, and the process of collecting such data could have the unintended consequence of compromising the doctor-patient therapeutic relationship. A requirement that the medical record include specific text could lead to documentation burden and overuse of standardized language that does not accurately reflect what has occurred in practice. In summary, these approaches to implementing a performance measure could seriously compromise the utility of the measure to influence practice and improve quality of care. The practicality of implementing measures based on this guideline may be improved, however, with future advancements in electronic medical records and natural language processing.

GUIDELINE IX. Documentation of the Psychiatric Evaluation

This guideline recommends that the initial psychiatric evaluation include documentation of the clinician's rationale for treatment selection, including a discussion of specific factors that influenced the treatment choice (statement 1). As described under "Expert Opinion Survey: Results," expert psychiatrists typically practice in accordance with this recommendation. The typical practices of other psychiatrists are unknown, but there may be variability. This variability could indicate a need to strengthen knowledge, improve training, and increase the time and attention that psychiatrists give to this aspect of documentation. Furthermore, there may be opportunities to improve quality in this area for patients seen by physicians in other fields of medicine. However, quality improvement activities that are derived from this recommendation must not oversimplify the process of documentation. As described under "Implementation," the breadth and depth of documentation will depend on the clinical circumstances and the complexity of decision making. Clinicians must use judgment to determine what level of documentation is appropriate for an individual patient. A performance measure, for example, that assesses for the presence or absence of specific text in the medical record could lead to documentation burden and overuse of standardized language that does not accurately reflect what has occurred in practice. Because of this practical challenge and potential burden, a performance measure derived from this recommendation is not recommended. The practicality of implementing a measure may be improved, however, with future advancements in electronic medical records and natural language processing.

Guideline Development Process

These guidelines were developed using a process intended to meet standards of the Institute of Medicine (2011). The process is fully described in a document available on the APA website: http://www.psychiatry.org/File%20Library/Practice/APA-Guideline-Development-Process--updated-2011-.pdf. Key elements of the development process included the following:

Management of Potential Conflicts of Interest

Work group members were required to disclose all potential conflicts of interest before appointment, before and during guideline development, and on publication. As described under "Disclosures," no member of the work group reported any conflicts of interest with his or her work on these guidelines. The two members of the Systematic Review Group also reported no conflicts of interest.

Work Group Composition

Because these guidelines addressed aspects of a psychiatric evaluation, the work group was composed of psychiatrists. However, some experts from other disciplines were included in the expert panel that was surveyed, as described under "Expert Opinion Data Collection." The work group was diverse and balanced with respect to their expertise as well as other characteristics, such as geographical location and demographic background. Methodological expertise (i.e., with respect to appraisal of strength of research evidence) was provided by the Systematic Review Group. A patient advocate (M.J.F.) was involved as an advisor during question formulation and draft review.

Expert Opinion Data Collection

An expert opinion survey was fielded to a panel of 1,738 experts in psychiatric evaluation and management. The response rate for the survey was 45.1% ($n=784$); 8.4% of the responses were partial, meaning that at least one of the eight sections of the survey was completed. Members of the panel were peer-nominated in 2011 by current and past APA work group members, chairs of academic departments of psychiatry and directors of psychiatry residency programs in the United States and Canada, and the APA Assembly. Survey questions were adapted from clinical questions developed by an APA expert work group and reviewed by a multidisciplinary group of stakeholders. The survey included questions to address which types of assessments improve identification of patients at risk for suicide and whether the experts typically perform such assessments in practice.

Nominators were asked to identify two types of experts to serve on the panel: researchers and clinicians. "Research experts" were defined as individuals who are making substantial contributions, via research or scholarly writing, to the area of psychiatric evaluation and management. "Clinical experts" were defined as individuals who have substantial clinical experience in the psychiatric evaluation of adults or an expert clinician whom the nominator might consult about an adult patient with a complex presentation. The panel was composed of approximately 70% clinical experts, 20% research experts, and 10% experts in both categories. Most of the panel members, 76.4%, were nominated once, 14.8% were nominated twice, and the remainder were nominated up to nine times. The majority of the panel members were contacted via email to complete the survey online; 1.8% were contacted via mail and 0.6% were not contacted because of lack of email or mailing address or inability to distinguish the intended nominee because of common names.

The composition of the portion of the panel who responded to the survey corresponds closely with that of the entire panel, within 0%–4% (i.e., in the number of times panel members were nominated and whether they were identified as clinical or research experts or both).

For each guideline, quantitative data from the survey are shown under "Review of Available Evidence." The survey also collected many free text comments, which were reviewed during development of the draft guidelines. Key themes from qualitative data have been incorporated into the implementation section of the guideline.

Systematic Review Methodology

These guidelines are based on a systematic search of available research evidence.

Systematic searches were conducted of the MEDLINE (PubMed), PsycINFO (EBSCOHost), and Cochrane (Wiley) databases. The search terms and limits used are available on request from the APA.

Search strategies were constructed that included a full range of topics related to psychiatric evaluation given the expected overlap in the retrieved literature for specific guideline questions. An initial search of MEDLINE was conducted in October 2010. This search yielded 250,981 articles. A second set of searches was conducted in October 2011. These searches yielded 32,895 articles in MEDLINE, 7,052 articles in PsycINFO, and 5,986 articles in the Cochrane database. All searches were done for the years from 1900 to the time of the search.

One individual (R.R.) screened 95,166 references from the 2010 search, spanning the years from 2005 to 2010. A second individual (L.F.) screened the 32,895 references from the 2011 search after duplicate articles from the different searches were eliminated. Included articles were those that pertained to a clinical trial (including a controlled or randomized trial), observational study, meta-analysis, or systematic review and were clinically relevant to psychiatric evaluation (i.e., relevant to any possible clinical question that might be addressed by potential APA practice guidelines). Excluded references included articles on nosology of psychiatric disorders, risk factors or associated features of specific disorders, potential etiologies of specific disorders, and course and prognosis of specific disorders.

A total of 5,073 articles met the broad inclusion criteria. These articles were screened by R.R. and L.F. for relevance to the clinical questions formulated for these guidelines and described under "Review of Supporting Research Evidence: Clinical Questions." The total number of studies that were agreed to have relevance to the PICOTS question for each guideline topic is as follows: 0 studies for Review of Psychiatric Symptoms, Trauma History, and Psychiatric Treatment History; 4 studies for Substance Use Assessment; 1 study for Assessment of Suicide Risk; 2 studies for Assessment of Risk for Aggressive Behaviors; 0 studies for Assessment of Cultural Factors; 3 studies for Assessment of Medical Health; 2 studies for Quantitative Assessment; 17 studies for Involvement of the Patient in Treatment Decision Making; and 0 studies for Documentation of the Psychiatric Evaluation.

An update of the literature search was conducted in September 2014 using the same databases and search strategies used for the October 2011 search. These searches in September 2014 yielded 8,521 additional articles in MEDLINE, 1,980 additional articles in PsycINFO, and 1,310 additional articles in the Cochrane database. After duplicates were eliminated, 11,644 abstracts were screened for relevance by two individuals (L.F., J.Y.). A total of 65 additional references met the broad inclusion criteria, and of these, 1 study was relevant to Quantitative Assessment.

For supporting sections of these guidelines (e.g., rationale, implementation), additional targeted searches of the literature were conducted to identify relevant references.

Rating the Strength of Supporting Research Evidence

"Strength of supporting research evidence" describes the level of confidence that findings from scientific observation and testing of an effect of an intervention reflect the true effect. Confidence is enhanced by factors such as rigorous study design and minimal potential for study bias. Three ratings are used: high, moderate, and low.

Ratings are determined by the Systematic Review Group, after assessment of available clinical trials across four primary domains: risk of bias, consistency of findings across studies, directness of the effect on a specific health outcome, and precision of the estimate of effect. These domains and the method used to evaluate them are described under "Systematic Review Methodology."

In accordance with the Methods Guide of the Agency for Healthcare Research and Quality (http://www.ncbi.nlm.nih.gov/books/NBK47095), the ratings are defined as follows:

- High (denoted by the letter *A*) = High confidence that the evidence reflects the true effect. Further research is very unlikely to change our confidence in the estimate of effect.
- Moderate (denoted by the letter *B*) = Moderate confidence that the evidence reflects the true effect. Further research may change our confidence in the estimate of effect and may change the estimate.
- Low (denoted by the letter *C*) = Low confidence that the evidence reflects the true effect. Further research is likely to change our confidence in the estimate of effect and is likely to change the estimate.

Rating the Strength of Recommendations

Each guideline statement is separately rated to indicate strength of recommendation and strength of supporting research evidence.

"Strength of recommendation" describes the level of confidence that potential benefits of an intervention outweigh potential harms. This level of confidence is informed by available evidence, which includes evidence from clinical trials as well as expert opinion and patient values and preferences. As described under "Guideline Development Process," the rating is a consensus judgment of the authors of the guideline and is endorsed by the APA Board of Trustees.

There are two possible ratings: recommendation or suggestion. These correspond to ratings of "strong" or "weak" (also termed "conditional") as defined under the GRADE method for rating recommendations in clinical practice guidelines (described in publications such as Guyatt et al. 2008 and others available on the website of the GRADE Working Group at http://gradeworkinggroup.org/index.htm). "Recommendation" (denoted by the numeral *1* after the guideline statement) indicates confidence that the benefits of the intervention clearly outweigh harms. "Suggestion" (denoted by the numeral *2* after the guideline statement) indicates uncertainty (i.e., the balance of benefits and harms is difficult to judge or either the benefits or the harms are unclear).

When a negative statement is made, ratings of strength of recommendation should be understood as meaning the inverse of the above (e.g., "recommendation" indicates confidence that harms clearly outweigh benefits).

When there is insufficient information to support a recommendation or a suggestion, a statement may be made that further research about the intervention is needed.

The work group determined ratings of strength of recommendation by the Delphi method—that is, through blind, iterative voting and discussion. In weighing potential benefits and harms, the group considered the strength of supporting research evidence, the results of the expert opinion survey, and their own clinical experiences and opinions. For recommendations, at least seven of the eight members of the group must have voted to "recommend" the intervention or assessment after three rounds of voting. If this level of consensus was not achieved, the work group could agree to make a "suggestion" rather than a recommendation. No suggestion or statement was made if three or more work group members voted "no statement." Differences of opinion within the group about ratings of strength of recommendation, if any, are described under "Review of Available Evidence."

External Review

These guidelines were made available for review in January 2014 by stakeholders, including the APA membership, scientific and clinical experts, allied organizations (including patient advocacy organizations), and the public. Eighty-seven individuals and 10 organizations submitted comments on one or more topics of the psychiatric evaluation guidelines. The work group reviewed and addressed all comments received. Revisions to ratings of strength of recommendation were determined by new Delphi voting.

Approval

These guidelines were submitted to the APA Board of Trustees for approval on December 14, 2014.

Glossary of Terms

Anxiety   The apprehensive anticipation of future danger or misfortune accompanied by a feeling of worry, distress, and/or somatic symptoms of tension (American Psychiatric Association 2013c).

Assessment   The process of obtaining information about a patient through any of a variety of methods, including face-to-face interview, review of medical records, physical examination (by the psychiatrist, another physician, or a medically trained clinician), diagnostic testing, or history taking from collateral sources.

Capacity for decision making   The ability of an individual, when faced with a specific clinical or treatment-related decision, "to communicate a choice, to understand the relevant information, to appreciate the medical consequences of the situation, and to reason about treatment choices" (Applebaum 2007, p. 1835).

Cultural factors related to social environment   The interface of cultural factors with the social environment may include, but is not limited to, an individual's family network, work place, religious group, community, or other psychosocial support network.

Culture   Systems of knowledge, concepts, rules, and practices that are learned and transmitted across generations. Culture includes language, religion and spirituality, family structures, life-cycle stages, ceremonial rituals, and customs, as well as moral and legal systems (American Psychiatric Association 2013c).

Hopelessness   Feeling of despair about the future out of the belief that there is no possibility of a solution to current problems or a positive outcome.

Impulsivity   Acting on the spur of the moment in response to immediate stimuli; acting on a momentary basis without a plan or consideration of outcomes; difficulty establishing and following plans; having a sense of urgency and exhibiting self-harming behavior under emotional distress (American Psychiatric Association 2013c).

Initial psychiatric evaluation   A comprehensive assessment of a patient that has the following aims: identify the reason that the patient is presenting for evaluation; establish rapport with the patient; understand the patient's background, relationships, current life circumstances, and strengths and vulnerabilities; establish whether the patient has a psychiatric condition; collect information needed to develop a differential diagnosis and clinical formulation; identify immediate concerns for patient safety; and develop an initial treatment plan or revise an existing plan in collaboration with the patient. Relevant information may be obtained by interviewing the patient, reviewing prior records, or obtaining collateral information from treating clinicians, family members, or others involved in the patient's life. Physical examination, laboratory studies, imaging, psychological or neuropsychological testing, or other assessments may also be included. The psychiatric evaluation may occur in a variety of settings, including inpatient or outpatient psychiatric settings and other medical settings. The evaluation is usually time intensive. The amount of time spent depends on the complexity of the problem, the clinical setting, and the patient's ability and willingness to cooperate with the assessment. Several meetings with the patient (and family or others) over time may be necessary. Psychiatrists may conduct other types of evaluations that have other goals (e.g., forensic evaluations) or that may be more focused and circumscribed than a psychiatric evaluation as defined here. These guidelines are not intended to address such evaluations.

Panic attacks   Discrete periods of sudden onset of intense fear or terror, often associated with feelings of impending doom. During these attacks there are symptoms such as shortness of breath or smothering sensations; palpitations, pounding heart, or accelerated heart rate; chest pain or discomfort; choking; and fear of going crazy or losing control (American Psychiatric Association 2013c).

Personal/cultural beliefs   Beliefs related to the patient's personal/cultural characteristics and identity, including but not limited to his or her beliefs about age, ethnicity, gender, race, religion, and sexuality.

Quantitative measures   Clinician- or patient-administered tests or scales that provide a numerical rating of features such as symptom severity, level of functioning, or quality of life and have been shown to be valid and reliable.

Stressor   Any emotional, physical, social, economic, or other factor that disrupts the normal physiological, cognitive, emotional, or behavioral balance of an individual (American Psychiatric Association 2013c).

Suicidal ideas   Thoughts of serving as the agent of one's own death.

Suicide attempt   A nonfatal, self-directed, potentially injurious behavior with any intent to die as a result of the behavior. A suicide attempt may or may not result in injury (Crosby et al. 2011). It may be aborted by the individual or interrupted by another individual.

Suicide intent   Subjective expectation and desire for a self-injurious act to end in death.

Suicide means   The instrument or object used to engage in self-inflicted injurious behavior with any intent to die as a result of the behavior.

Suicide method   The mechanism used to engage in self-inflicted injurious behavior with any intent to die as a result of the behavior.

Suicide plan   Delineation of the method, means, time, place, or other details for engaging in self-inflicted injurious behavior with any intent to die as a result of the behavior.

Suicide   Death caused by self-directed injurious behavior with any intent to die as a result of the behavior (Crosby et al. 2011).

Therapeutic alliance   A characteristic of the relationship between the patient and clinician that describes the sense of collaboration in pursuing therapeutic goals as well as the patient's sense of attachment to the clinician and perception of whether the clinician is helpful (Gabbard 2009).

Trauma history   A history of events in the patient's life with the potential to have been emotionally traumatic, including but not limited to exposure to actual or threatened death, serious injury, illness, or sexual violence. Exposure may occur through direct experience or by observing an event in person or through technology (e.g., television, audio/video recording) or by learning of an event that occurred to a close family member or close friend. Trauma could also include early adversity, neglect, maltreatment, emotional abuse, physical abuse, or sexual abuse occurring in childhood; exposure to natural or man-made disasters; exposure to combat situations; being a victim of a violent crime; involvement in a serious motor vehicle accident; or having serious or painful or prolonged medical experiences (e.g., intensive care unit stay).

References

Abderhalden C, Needham I, Dassen T, et al: Structured risk assessment and violence in acute psychiatric wards: randomised controlled trial. Br J Psychiatry 193(1):44–50, 2008 18700217 *

Abdullah T, Brown TL: Mental illness stigma and ethnocultural beliefs, values, and norms: an integrative review. Clin Psychol Rev 31(6):934–948, 2011 21683671

Agabio R, Marras P, Gessa GL, Carpiniello B: Alcohol use disorders, and at-risk drinking in patients affected by a mood disorder, in Cagliari, Italy: sensitivity and specificity of different questionnaires. Alcohol Alcohol 42(6):575–581, 2007 17766313 *

Agency for Healthcare Research and Quality: Methods Guide for Effectiveness and Comparative Effectiveness Reviews. AHRQ Publication No. 10(14)-EHC063-EF. Rockville, MD, Agency for Healthcare Research and Quality, January 2014. Available at: http://www.effectivehealthcare.ahrq.gov/ehc/products/60/318/CER-Methods-Guide-140109.pdf. Accessed May 24, 2015.

Allen JG, Frueh BC, Ellis TE, et al: Integrating outcomes assessment and research into clinical care in inpatient adult psychiatric treatment. Bull Menninger Clin 73(4):259–295, 2009 20025425

Althof SE, Rosen RC, Perelman MA, Rubio-Aurioles E: Standard operating procedures for taking a sexual history. J Sex Med 10(1):26–35, 2013 22970717

AMA Council on Ethical and Judicial Affairs: Code of Medical Ethics of the American Medical Association, 2012--2013. Chicago, IL, American Medical Association, 2012

American College of Obstetricians and Gynecologists, Committee on Health Care for Underserved Women, Committee on Obstetric Practice: Committee opinion no. 471: Smoking cessation during pregnancy. Obstet Gynecol 116(5):1241–1244, 2010 20966731

American College of Obstetricians and Gynecologists, Committee on Health Care for Underserved Women: Committee opinion no. 496: At-risk drinking and alcohol dependence: obstetric and gynecologic implications. Obstet Gynecol 118(2 Pt 1):383–388, 2011 21775870

American College of Obstetricians and Gynecologists, Committee on Health Care for Underserved Women; American Society of Addiction Medicine: ACOG Committee Opinion No. 524: Opioid abuse, dependence, and addiction in pregnancy. Obstet Gynecol 119(5):1070–1076, 2012 22525931

American Psychiatric Association: Cultural formulation, in Diagnostic and Statistical Manual of Mental Disorders, 5th Edition. Arlington, VA, American Psychiatric Association, 2013a, pp 749–759

American Psychiatric Association: Diagnostic and Statistical Manual of Mental Disorders, 5th Edition. Arlington, VA, American Psychiatric Publishing, 2013b

American Psychiatric Association: Glossary of technical terms, in Diagnostic and Statistical Manual of Mental Disorders, 5th Edition. Arlington, VA, American Psychiatric Association, 2013c, pp 817–831

Andrews JC, Schünemann HJ, Oxman AD, et al: GRADE guidelines: 15. Going from evidence to recommendation-determinants of a recommendation's direction and strength. J Clin Epidemiol 66(7):726–735, 2013 23570745

Angermeyer MC, Dietrich S: Public beliefs about and attitudes towards people with mental illness: a review of population studies. Acta Psychiatr Scand 113(3):163–179, 2006 16466402

Appelbaum PS: Clinical practice. Assessment of patients' competence to consent to treatment. N Engl J Med 357(18):1834–1840, 2007 17978292

Arbuckle MR, Weinberg M, Kistler SC, et al: A curriculum in measurement-based care: screening and monitoring of depression in a psychiatric resident clinic. Acad Psychiatry 37(5):317–320, 2013 24026369

Arsenault-Lapierre G, Kim C, Turecki G: Psychiatric diagnoses in 3275 suicides: a meta-analysis. BMC Psychiatry 4:37, 2004 15527502

References to supporting research evidence are denoted by *.

Assessment and Management of Risk for Suicide Working Group: VA/DoD Clinical Practice Guideline for Assessment and Management of Patients at Risk for Suicide. Version 1.0. Washington, DC, Department of Veterans Affairs, Department of Defense, June 2013

Balshem H, Helfand M, Schünemann HJ, et al: GRADE guidelines: 3. Rating the quality of evidence. J Clin Epidemiol 64(4):401–406, 2011 21208779

Barber ME, Marzuk PM, Leon AC, Portera L: Aborted suicide attempts: a new classification of suicidal behavior. Am J Psychiatry 155(3):385–389, 1998 9501750

Barry KL, Milner K, Blow FC, et al: Screening psychiatric emergency department patients with major mental illnesses for at-risk drinking. Psychiatr Serv 57(7):1039–1042, 2006 16816292 *

Bartsch DA, Shern DL, Feinberg LE, et al: Screening CMHC outpatients for physical illness. Hosp Community Psychiatry 41(7):786–790, 1990 2365313 *

Bate L, Hutchinson A, Underhill J, Maskrey N: How clinical decisions are made. Br J Clin Pharmacol 74(4):614–620, 2012 22738381

Bauer AM, Alegría M: Impact of patient language proficiency and interpreter service use on the quality of psychiatric care: a systematic review. Psychiatr Serv 61(8):765–773, 2010 20675834

Bauer AM, Chen CN, Alegría M: English language proficiency and mental health service use among Latino and Asian Americans with mental disorders. Med Care 48(12):1097–1104, 2010 21063226

Baxter D, Appleby L: Case register study of suicide risk in mental disorders. Br J Psychiatry 175:322–326, 1999 10789297

Beauchamp TL: Informed consent: its history, meaning, and present challenges. Camb Q Healthc Ethics 20(4):515–523, 2011 21843382

Beauchamp TL, Childress JF: Principles of Biomedical Ethics, 7th Edition. New York, Oxford University Press, 2012

Bertolote JM, Fleischmann A, De Leo D, Wasserman D: Psychiatric diagnoses and suicide: revisiting the evidence. Crisis 25(4):147–155, 2004 15580849

Bickman L, Kelley SD, Breda C, et al: Effects of routine feedback to clinicians on mental health outcomes of youths: results of a randomized trial. Psychiatr Serv 62(12):1423–1429, 2011 22193788

Borges G, Nock MK, Haro Abad JM, et al: Twelve-month prevalence of and risk factors for suicide attempts in the World Health Organization World Mental Health Surveys. J Clin Psychiatry 71(12):1617–1628, 2010 20816034

Boswell JF, Kraus DR, Miller SD, Lambert MJ: Implementing routine outcome monitoring in clinical practice: Benefits, challenges, and solutions. Psychother Res 25(1):6–19, 2015 23885809

Brahm NC, Yeager LL, Fox MD, et al: Commonly prescribed medications and potential false-positive urine drug screens. Am J Health Syst Pharm 67(16):1344–1350, 2010 20689123

Brito JP, Domecq JP, Murad MH, et al: The Endocrine Society guidelines: when the confidence cart goes before the evidence horse. J Clin Endocrinol Metab 98(8):3246–3252, 2013 23783104

Bromet EJ, Kotov R, Fochtmann LJ, et al: Diagnostic shifts during the decade following first admission for psychosis. Am J Psychiatry 168(11):1186–1194, 2011 21676994

Brown GK, Beck AT, Steer RA, Grisham JR: Risk factors for suicide in psychiatric outpatients: a 20-year prospective study. J Consult Clin Psychol 68(3):371–377, 2000 10883553

Brownlie K, Schneider C, Culliford R, et al: Medication reconciliation by a pharmacy technician in a mental health assessment unit. Int J Clin Pharm 36(2):303–309, 2014

Buchanan A, Binder R, Norko M, Swartz M: Psychiatric violence risk assessment. Am J Psychiatry 169(3):340, 2012 22407122

Buchkremer G, Klingberg S, Holle R, et al: Psychoeducational psychotherapy for schizophrenic patients and their key relatives or care-givers: results of a 2-year follow-up. Acta Psychiatr Scand 96(6):483–491, 1997 9421346 *

Bush K, Kivlahan DR, McDonell MB, et al: The AUDIT alcohol consumption questions (AUDIT-C): an effective brief screening test for problem drinking. Ambulatory Care Quality Improvement Project (ACQUIP). Alcohol Use Disorders Identification Test. Arch Intern Med 158(16):1789–1795, 1998 9738608

Carlson EB, Smith SR, Palmieri PA, et al: Development and validation of a brief self-report measure of trauma exposure: the Trauma History Screen. Psychol Assess 23(2):463–477, 2011 21517189

Carroll R, Metcalfe C, Gunnell D: Hospital presenting self-harm and risk of fatal and non-fatal repetition: systematic review and meta-analysis. PLoS ONE 9(2):e89944, 2014 24587141

Cavanagh JT, Carson AJ, Sharpe M, Lawrie SM: Psychological autopsy studies of suicide: a systematic review. Psychol Med 33(3):395–405, 2003 12701661

Centers for Medicare & Medicaid Services: Evaluation and Management Services Guide. Baltimore, MD, Centers for Medicare & Medicaid Services, November 2014. Available at: http://www.cms.gov/Outreach-and-Education/Medicare-Learning-Network-MLN/MLNProducts/downloads/eval_mgmt_serv_guide-ICN006764.pdf. Accessed May 25, 2015.

The APA Practice Guidelines for the Psychiatric Evaluation of Adults, Third Edition

Chafetz L, White MC, Collins-Bride G, et al: Predictors of physical functioning among adults with severe mental illness. Psychiatr Serv 57(2):225–231, 2006 16452700

Chang CK, Hayes RD, Broadbent M, et al: All-cause mortality among people with serious mental illness (SMI), substance use disorders, and depressive disorders in southeast London: a cohort study. BMC Psychiatry 10:77, 2010 20920287

Charles C, Gafni A, Whelan T, O'Brien MA: Cultural influences on the physician-patient encounter: the case of shared treatment decision-making. Patient Educ Couns 63(3):262–267, 2006 17000073

Chewning B, Bylund CL, Shah B, et al: Patient preferences for shared decisions: a systematic review. Patient Educ Couns 86(1):9–18, 2012 21474265

Chung H, Duffy FF, Katzelnick DJ, et al: Sustaining practice change one year after completion of the national depression management leadership initiative. Psychiatr Serv 64(7):703–706, 2013 23821170

Chwastiak LA, Rosenheck RA, Desai R, Kazis LE: Association of psychiatric illness and all-cause mortality in the National Department of Veterans Affairs Health Care System. Psychosom Med 72(8):817–822, 2010 20639387

Cohen AN, Drapalski AL, Glynn SM, et al: Preferences for family involvement in care among consumers with serious mental illness. Psychiatr Serv 64(3):257–263, 2013 23242515

Coid J, Yang M, Roberts A, et al: Violence and psychiatric morbidity in a national household population—a report from the British Household Survey. Am J Epidemiol 164(12):1199–1208, 2006 17032695

Compton WM, Thomas YF, Stinson FS, Grant BF: Prevalence, correlates, disability, and comorbidity of DSM-IV drug abuse and dependence in the United States: results from the national epidemiologic survey on alcohol and related conditions. Arch Gen Psychiatry 64(5):566–576, 2007 17485608

Conner KR, Duberstein PR, Conwell Y, et al: Psychological vulnerability to completed suicide: a review of empirical studies. Suicide Life Threat Behav 31(4):367–385, 2001 11775713

Cornaggia CM, Beghi M, Pavone F, Barale F: Aggression in psychiatry wards: a systematic review. Psychiatry Res 189(1):10–20, 2011 21236497

Coryell W, Young EA: Clinical predictors of suicide in primary major depressive disorder. J Clin Psychiatry 66(4):412–417, 2005 15816781

Council of Medical Specialty Societies: Principles for the Development of Specialty Society Clinical Guidelines. Chicago, IL, Council of Medical Specialty Societies, 2012

Coverdale JH, Turbott SH: Sexual and physical abuse of chronically ill psychiatric outpatients compared with a matched sample of medical outpatients. J Nerv Ment Dis 188(7):440–445, 2000 10919703

Covey J: A meta-analysis of the effects of presenting treatment benefits in different formats. Med Decis Making 27(5):638–654, 2007 17873250

Crosby AE, Ortega L, Melanson C: Self-Directed Violence Surveillance: Uniform Definitions and Recommended Data Elements, Version 1.0. Atlanta, GA, Centers for Disease Control and Prevention, National Center for Injury Prevention and Control, February 2011. Available at: http://www.cdc.gov/violenceprevention/pdf/self-directed-violence-a.pdf. Accessed May 25, 2015.

Croskerry P, Singhal G, Mamede S: Cognitive debiasing 1: origins of bias and theory of debiasing. BMJ Qual Saf 22(Suppl 2):ii58–ii64, 2013 23882089

Cusack CM, Hripcsak G, Bloomrosen M, et al: The future state of clinical data capture and documentation: a report from AMIA's 2011 Policy Meeting. J Am Med Inform Assoc 20(1):134–140, 2013 22962195

Cusack KJ, Frueh BC, Brady KT: Trauma history screening in a community mental health center. Psychiatr Serv 55(2):157–162, 2004 14762240

Dack C, Ross J, Papadopoulos C, et al: A review and meta-analysis of the patient factors associated with psychiatric in-patient aggression. Acta Psychiatr Scand 127(4):255–268, 2013 23289890

David AS, Fleminger S, Kopelman MD, et al (eds): Lishman's Organic Psychiatry: A Textbook of Neuropsychiatry, 4th Edition. Oxford, UK, Wiley-Blackwell, 2009

Deegan PE, Drake RE: Shared decision making and medication management in the recovery process. Psychiatr Serv 57(11):1636–1639, 2006 17085613

Degmecić D, Pozgain I, Filaković P: Psychoeducation and compliance in the treatment of patients with schizophrenia. Coll Antropol 31(4):1111–1115, 2007 18217468 *

Dening KH, Jones L, Sampson EL: Advance care planning for people with dementia: a review. Int Psychogeriatr 23(10):1535–1551, 2011 21867597

Dickerson FB, Brown CH, Daumit GL, et al: Health status of individuals with serious mental illness. Schizophr Bull 32(3):584–589, 2006a 16469943 (corrected in Schizophr Bull 33[5]:1257, 2007)

Dickerson FB, Brown CH, Kreyenbuhl JA, et al: Obesity among individuals with serious mental illness. Acta Psychiatr Scand 113(4):306–313, 2006b 16638075

Diener E, Emmons RA, Larsen RJ, Griffin S: The Satisfaction With Life Scale. J Pers Assess 49(1):71–75, 1985 16367493

Dixon LB, Glynn SM, Cohen AN, et al: Outcomes of a brief program, REORDER, to promote consumer recovery and family involvement in care. Psychiatr Serv 65(1):116–120, 2014 24177229

Djulbegovic B, Trikalinos TA, Roback J, et al: Impact of quality of evidence on the strength of recommendations: an empirical study. BMC Health Serv Res 9:120, 2009 19622148

Douglas KS, Guy LS, Hart SD: Psychosis as a risk factor for violence to others: a meta-analysis. Psychol Bull 135(5):679–706, 2009 19702378

Doyle M, Dolan M: Predicting community violence from patients discharged from mental health services. Br J Psychiatry 189:520–526, 2006 17139036

Doyle M, Carter S, Shaw J, Dolan M: Predicting community violence from patients discharged from acute mental health units in England. Soc Psychiatry Psychiatr Epidemiol 47(4):627–637, 2012 21390510

Drake RE, Deegan PE: Shared decision making is an ethical imperative. Psychiatr Serv 60(8):1007, 2009 19648184

Drenth-van Maanen AC, Spee J, van Hensbergen L, et al: Structured history taking of medication use reveals iatrogenic harm due to discrepancies in medication histories in hospital and pharmacy records. J Am Geriatr Soc 59(10):1976–1977, 2011 22091519

Druss BG, Zhao L, Von Esenwein S, et al: Understanding excess mortality in persons with mental illness: 17-year follow up of a nationally representative US survey. Med Care 49(6):599–604, 2011 21577183

Duffy FF, Chung H, Trivedi M, et al: Systematic use of patient-rated depression severity monitoring: is it helpful and feasible in clinical psychiatry? Psychiatr Serv 59(10):1148–1154, 2008 18832500

Dunlop BW, Kelley ME, Mletzko TC, et al: Depression beliefs, treatment preference, and outcomes in a randomized trial for major depressive disorder. J Psychiatr Res 46(3):375–381, 2012 22118808

Edwards AG, Naik G, Ahmed H, et al: Personalised risk communication for informed decision making about taking screening tests. Cochrane Database Syst Rev 2:CD001865, 2013 23450534

Elbogen EB, Johnson SC: The intricate link between violence and mental disorder: results from the National Epidemiologic Survey on Alcohol and Related Conditions. Arch Gen Psychiatry 66(2):152–161, 2009 19188537

Elbogen EB, Van Dorn RA, Swanson JW, et al: Treatment engagement and violence risk in mental disorders. Br J Psychiatry 189:354–360, 2006 17012659

Elbogen EB, Van Dorn R, Swanson JW, et al: Effectively implementing psychiatric advance directives to promote Self-determination of treatment among people with mental illness. Psychol Public Policy Law 13(4): 2007 24198456

Elwyn G, Frosch D, Thomson R, et al: Shared decision making: a model for clinical practice. J Gen Intern Med 27(10):1361–1367, 2012 22618581

Embi PJ, Weir C, Efthimiadis EN, et al: Computerized provider documentation: findings and implications of a multisite study of clinicians and administrators. J Am Med Inform Assoc 20(4):718–726, 2013 23355462

Epstein RM, Gramling RE: What is shared in shared decision making? Complex decisions when the evidence is unclear. Med Care Res Rev 70(1)(Suppl):94S–112S, 2013 23035055

Epstein RM, Peters E: Beyond information: exploring patients' preferences. JAMA 302(2):195–197, 2009 19584351

Eriksson A, Romelsjö A, Stenbacka M, Tengström A: Early risk factors for criminal offending in schizophrenia: a 35-year longitudinal cohort study. Soc Psychiatry Psychiatr Epidemiol 46(9):925–932, 2011 20607212

Falk O, Wallinius M, Lundström S, et al: The 1% of the population accountable for 63% of all violent crime convictions. Soc Psychiatry Psychiatr Epidemiol 49(4):559–571, 2014 24173408

Fazel S, Gulati G, Linsell L, et al: Schizophrenia and violence: systematic review and meta-analysis. PLoS Med 6(8):e1000120, 2009a 19668362

Fazel S, Philipson J, Gardiner L, et al: Neurological disorders and violence: a systematic review and meta-analysis with a focus on epilepsy and traumatic brain injury. J Neurol 256(10):1591–1602, 2009b 19353216

Fazel S, Lichtenstein P, Grann M, et al: Bipolar disorder and violent crime: new evidence from population-based longitudinal studies and systematic review. Arch Gen Psychiatry 67(9):931–938, 2010 20819987

Fazel S, Singh JP, Doll H, Grann M: Use of risk assessment instruments to predict violence and antisocial behaviour in 73 samples involving 24 827 people: systematic review and meta-analysis. BMJ 345:e4692, 2012 22833604

Feighner JP, Robins E, Guze SB, et al: Diagnostic criteria for use in psychiatric research. Arch Gen Psychiatry 26(1):57–63, 1972 5009428

Fellinger J, Holzinger D, Pollard R: Mental health of deaf people. Lancet 379(9820):1037–1044, 2012 22423884

Fernandez A, Schillinger D, Warton EM, et al: Language barriers, physician-patient language concordance, and glycemic control among insured Latinos with diabetes: the Diabetes Study of Northern California (DISTANCE). J Gen Intern Med 26(2):170–176, 2011 20878497

Ferrando SJ, Levenson JL, Owen JA (eds): Clinical Manual of Psychopharmacology in the Medically Ill. Washington, DC, American Psychiatric Publishing, 2010

Fiore MC, Jaén CR, Baker TB, et al: Treating Tobacco Use and Dependence: 2008 Update. Clinical Practice Guideline. Rockville, MD, U.S. Department of Health and Human Services. Public Health Service, May 2008

Fitzgerald RJ: Medication errors: the importance of an accurate drug history. Br J Clin Pharmacol 67(6):671–675, 2009 19594536

Fok ML, Hayes RD, Chang CK, et al: Life expectancy at birth and all-cause mortality among people with personality disorder. J Psychosom Res 73(2):104–107, 2012 22789412

Freeman MP, Fava M, Lake J, et al: Complementary and alternative medicine in major depressive disorder: the American Psychiatric Association Task Force report. J Clin Psychiatry 71(6):669–681, 2010 20573326

Friedberg MW, Van Busum K, Wexler R, et al: A demonstration of shared decision making in primary care highlights barriers to adoption and potential remedies. Health Aff (Millwood) 32(2):268–275, 2013 23381519

Frosch DL, May SG, Rendle KA, et al: Authoritarian physicians and patients' fear of being labeled "difficult" among key obstacles to shared decision making. Health Aff (Millwood) 31(5):1030–1038, 2012 22566443

Frueh BC, Knapp RG, Cusack KJ, et al: Patients' reports of traumatic or harmful experiences within the psychiatric setting. Psychiatr Serv 56(9):1123–1133, 2005 16148328

Gabbard GO: Techniques of psychodynamic psychotherapy, in Textbook of Psychotherapeutic Treatments. Edited by Gabbard GO. Washington, DC, American Psychiatric Publishing, 2009, pp 43–67

Gadermann AM, Alonso J, Vilagut G, et al: Comorbidity and disease burden in the National Comorbidity Survey Replication (NCS-R). Depress Anxiety 29(9):797–806, 2012 22585578

Gany F, Leng J, Shapiro E, et al: Patient satisfaction with different interpreting methods: a randomized controlled trial. J Gen Intern Med 22(Suppl 2):312–318, 2007 17957417

Gelhorn HL, Sexton CC, Classi PM: Patient preferences for treatment of major depressive disorder and the impact on health outcomes: a systematic review. Prim Care Companion CNS Disord 13(5), pii 2011 22295273

Geulayov G, Gunnell D, Holmen TL, Metcalfe C: The association of parental fatal and non-fatal suicidal behaviour with offspring suicidal behaviour and depression: a systematic review and meta-analysis. Psychol Med 42(8):1567–1580, 2012 22129460

Goldberg JF, Ernst CL: Managing the Side Effects of Psychotropic Medications. Washington, DC, American Psychiatric Publishing, 2012

Goldberg RW, Kreyenbuhl JA, Medoff DR, et al: Quality of diabetes care among adults with serious mental illness. Psychiatr Serv 58(4):536–543, 2007 17412857

Goldstein RB, Black DW, Nasrallah A, Winokur G: The prediction of suicide: sensitivity, specificity, and predictive value of a multivariate model applied to suicide among 1906 patients with affective disorders. Arch Gen Psychiatry 48(5):418–422, 1991 2021294

Gone JP, Trimble JE: American Indian and Alaska Native mental health: diverse perspectives on enduring disparities. Annu Rev Clin Psychol 8:131–160, 2012 22149479

Grant BF, Hasin DS, Chou SP, et al: Nicotine dependence and psychiatric disorders in the United States: results from the national epidemiologic survey on alcohol and related conditions. Arch Gen Psychiatry 61(11):1107–1115, 2004 15520358

Gray R: Does patient education enhance compliance with clozapine? A preliminary investigation. J Psychiatr Ment Health Nurs 7(3):285–286, 2000 11249323 *

Grote NK, Swartz HA, Geibel SL, et al: A randomized controlled trial of culturally relevant, brief interpersonal psychotherapy for perinatal depression. Psychiatr Serv 60(3):313–321, 2009 19252043

Guyatt G, Gutterman D, Baumann MH, et al: Grading strength of recommendations and quality of evidence in clinical guidelines: report from an American College of Chest Physicians task force. Chest 129(1):174–181, 2006 16424429

Guyatt GH, Oxman AD, Kunz R, et al; GRADE Working Group: Going from evidence to recommendations. BMJ 336(7652):1049–1051, 2008 18467413

Guyatt G, Eikelboom JW, Akl EA, et al: A guide to GRADE guidelines for the readers of JTH. J Thromb Haemost 11(8):1603–1608, 2013 23773710

Haklai Z, Goldberger N, Stein N, et al: The mortality risk among persons with psychiatric hospitalizations. Isr J Psychiatry Relat Sci 48(4):230–239, 2011 22572086

Hall RC, Gardner ER, Popkin MK, et al: Unrecognized physical illness prompting psychiatric admission: a prospective study. Am J Psychiatry 138(5):629–635, 1981 7235058 *

Hall-Lipsy EA, Chisholm-Burns MA: Pharmacotherapeutic disparities: racial, ethnic, and sex variations in medication treatment. Am J Health Syst Pharm 67(6):462–468, 2010 20208053

Hamann J, Langer B, Winkler V, et al: Shared decision making for in-patients with schizophrenia. Acta Psychiatr Scand 114(4):265–273, 2006 16968364 *

Hamann J, Cohen R, Leucht S, et al: Shared decision making and long-term outcome in schizophrenia treatment. J Clin Psychiatry 68(7):992–997, 2007 17685733 *

Hamilton M: A rating scale for depression. J Neurol Neurosurg Psychiatry 23:56–62, 1960 14399272

Hammond KW, Efthimiadis EN, Weir CR, et al: Initial steps toward validating and measuring the quality of computerized provider documentation. AMIA Annual Symposium Proceedings, November 13, 2010, pp 271–275

Haney EM, O'Neil ME, Carson S, et al: Suicide Risk Factors and Risk Assessment Tools: A Systematic Review. VA-ESP Project #05-225. Washington, DC, Department of Veterans Affairs, March 2012

Harding KJ, Rush AJ, Arbuckle M, et al: Measurement-based care in psychiatric practice: a policy framework for implementation. J Clin Psychiatry 72(8):1136–1143, 2011 21295000

Harford TC, Yi HY, Grant BF: Other- and self-directed forms of violence and their relationships to DSM-IV substance use and other psychiatric disorders in a national survey of adults. Compr Psychiatry 54(7):731–739, 2013 23587529

Harris EC, Barraclough B: Suicide as an outcome for mental disorders. A meta-analysis. Br J Psychiatry 170:205–228, 1997 9229027

Hasin DS, Stinson FS, Ogburn E, Grant BF: Prevalence, correlates, disability, and comorbidity of DSM-IV alcohol abuse and dependence in the United States: results from the National Epidemiologic Survey on Alcohol and Related Conditions. Arch Gen Psychiatry 64(7):830–842, 2007 17606817

Haueis P, Greil W, Huber M, et al: Evaluation of drug interactions in a large sample of psychiatric inpatients: a data interface for mass analysis with clinical decision support software. Clin Pharmacol Ther 90(4):588–596, 2011 21866099

Hawton K, van Heeringen K: Suicide. Lancet 373(9672):1372–1381, 2009 19376453

Hawton K, Saunders K, Topiwala A, Haw C: Psychiatric disorders in patients presenting to hospital following self-harm: a systematic review. J Affect Disord 151(3):821–830, 2013 24091302

Hayes RD, Chang CK, Fernandes AC, et al: Functional status and all-cause mortality in serious mental illness. PLoS ONE 7(9):e44613, 2012 22970266

Hazlehurst JM, Armstrong MJ, Sherlock M, et al: A comparative quality assessment of evidence-based clinical guidelines in endocrinology. Clin Endocrinol (Oxf) 78(2):183–190, 2013 22624723

Heatherton TF, Kozlowski LT, Frecker RC, Fagerström KO: The Fagerström Test for Nicotine Dependence: a revision of the Fagerström Tolerance Questionnaire. Br J Addict 86(9):1119–1127, 1991 1932883

Henneman PL, Mendoza R, Lewis RJ: Prospective evaluation of emergency department medical clearance. Ann Emerg Med 24(4):672–677, 1994 7619102 *

Hill KP, Chang G: Brief screening instruments for risky drinking in the outpatient psychiatry clinic. Am J Addict 16(3):222–226, 2007 17612827 *

Honkonen H, Mattila AK, Lehtinen K, et al: Mortality of Finnish acute psychiatric hospital patients. Soc Psychiatry Psychiatr Epidemiol 43(8):660–666, 2008 18478169

Hornung WP, Kieserg A, Feldmann R, Buchkremer G: Psychoeducational training for schizophrenic patients: background, procedure and empirical findings. Patient Educ Couns 29(3):257–268, 1996 9006241 *

Hornung WP, Klingberg S, Feldmann R, et al: Collaboration with drug treatment by schizophrenic patients with and without psychoeducational training: results of a 1-year follow-up. Acta Psychiatr Scand 97(3):213–219, 1998 9543310 *

Hovens JG, Giltay EJ, Wiersma JE, et al: Impact of childhood life events and trauma on the course of depressive and anxiety disorders. Acta Psychiatr Scand 126(3):198–207, 2012 22268708

Høye A, Jacobsen BK, Hansen V: Sex differences in mortality of admitted patients with personality disorders in North Norway—a prospective register study. BMC Psychiatry 13(1):317, 2013 24279812

Huang B, Dawson DA, Stinson FS, et al: Prevalence, correlates, and comorbidity of nonmedical prescription drug use and drug use disorders in the United States: Results of the National Epidemiologic Survey on Alcohol and Related Conditions. J Clin Psychiatry 67(7):1062–1073, 2006 16889449

Iacoviello BM, McCarthy KS, Barrett MS, et al: Treatment preferences affect the therapeutic alliance: implications for randomized controlled trials. J Consult Clin Psychol 75(1):194–198, 2007 17295580 *

Ilgen MA, Kleinberg F, Ignacio RV, et al: Noncancer pain conditions and risk of suicide. JAMA Psychiatry 70(7):692–697, 2013 23699975

Institute of Medicine: Clinical Practice Guidelines We Can Trust. Washington, DC, National Academies Press, 2011

Jimenez DE, Bartels SJ, Cardenas V, et al: Cultural beliefs and mental health treatment preferences of ethnically diverse older adult consumers in primary care. Am J Geriatr Psychiatry 20(6):533–542, 2012 21992942

Jobes DA: The Collaborative Assessment and Management of Suicidality (CAMS): an evolving evidence-based clinical approach to suicidal risk. Suicide Life Threat Behav 42(6):640–653, 2012 22971238

Jonas DE, Garbutt JC, Amick HR, et al: Behavioral counseling after screening for alcohol misuse in primary care: a systematic review and meta-analysis for the U.S. Preventive Services Task Force. Ann Intern Med 157(9):645–654, 2012a 23007881

Jonas DE, Garbutt JC, Brown JM, et al: Screening, Behavioral Counseling, and Referral in Primary Care to Reduce Alcohol Misuse. Comparative Effectiveness Reviews No 64. (Report No 12-EHC055-EF). Rockville, MD, Agency for Healthcare Research and Quality, 2012b

Karliner LS, Jacobs EA, Chen AH, Mutha S: Do professional interpreters improve clinical care for patients with limited English proficiency? A systematic review of the literature. Health Serv Res 42(2):727–754, 2007 17362215

Katzelnick DJ, Duffy FF, Chung H, et al: Depression outcomes in psychiatric clinical practice: using a self-rated measure of depression severity. Psychiatr Serv 62(8):929–935, 2011 21807833

Kessler RC, Chiu WT, Demler O, et al: Prevalence, severity, and comorbidity of 12-month DSM-IV disorders in the National Comorbidity Survey Replication. Arch Gen Psychiatry 62(6):617–627, 2005 15939839

Kessler RC, Wang PS: The descriptive epidemiology of commonly occurring mental disorders in the United States. Annu Rev Public Health 29:115–129, 2008 18348707

Kilbourne AM, McCarthy JF, Welsh D, Blow F: Recognition of co-occurring medical conditions among patients with serious mental illness. J Nerv Ment Dis 194(8):598–602, 2006 16909068

Kilbourne AM, Welsh D, McCarthy JF, et al: Quality of care for cardiovascular disease-related conditions in patients with and without mental disorders. J Gen Intern Med 23(10):1628–1633, 2008 18626722

Kim G, Aguado Loi CX, Chiriboga DA, et al: Limited English proficiency as a barrier to mental health service use: a study of Latino and Asian immigrants with psychiatric disorders. J Psychiatr Res 45(1):104–110, 2011 20537658

King EA, Baldwin DS, Sinclair JM, et al: The Wessex Recent In-Patient Suicide Study, 1. Case-control study of 234 recently discharged psychiatric patient suicides. Br J Psychiatry 178:531–536, 2001 11388969

Kisely S, Sadek J, MacKenzie A, et al: Excess cancer mortality in psychiatric patients. Can J Psychiatry 53(11):753–761, 2008 19087469

Kisely S, Quek LH, Pais J, et al: Advanced dental disease in people with severe mental illness: systematic review and meta-analysis. Br J Psychiatry 199(3):187–193, 2011 21881097

Klein E, Rosenberg J, Rosenberg S: Whose treatment is it anyway? The role of consumer preferences in mental health care. Am J Psychiatr Rehabil 10(1):65–80, 2007

Knops AM, Legemate DA, Goossens A, et al: Decision aids for patients facing a surgical treatment decision: a systematic review and meta-analysis. Ann Surg 257(5):860–866, 2013 23470574

Kocsis JH, Leon AC, Markowitz JC, et al: Patient preference as a moderator of outcome for chronic forms of major depressive disorder treated with nefazodone, cognitive behavioral analysis system of psychotherapy, or their combination. J Clin Psychiatry 70(3):354–361, 2009 19192474

Kon AA: Difficulties in judging patient preferences for shared decision-making. J Med Ethics 38(12):719–720, 2012 23180253

Kraemer HC, Kazdin AE, Offord DR, et al: Coming to terms with the terms of risk. Arch Gen Psychiatry 54(4):337–343, 1997 9107150

Kroenke K, Spitzer RL, Williams JB: The PHQ-9: validity of a brief depression severity measure. J Gen Intern Med 16(9):606–613, 2001 11556941

Kwan BM, Dimidjian S, Rizvi SL: Treatment preference, engagement, and clinical improvement in pharmacotherapy versus psychotherapy for depression. Behav Res Ther 48(8):799–804, 2010 20462569

Kwan JL, Lo L, Sampson M, Shojania KG: Medication reconciliation during transitions of care as a patient safety strategy: a systematic review. Ann Intern Med 158(5 Pt 2):397–403, 2013 23460096

Lagomasino IT, Dwight-Johnson M, Miranda J, et al: Disparities in depression treatment for Latinos and site of care. Psychiatr Serv 56(12):1517–1523, 2005 16339612

Large M, Ryan C, Nielssen O: The validity and utility of risk assessment for inpatient suicide. Australas Psychiatry 19(6):507–512, 2011a 22077302

Large MM, Ryan CJ, Singh SP, et al: The predictive value of risk categorization in schizophrenia. Harv Rev Psychiatry 19(1):25–33, 2011b 21250894

Large M, Smith G, Sharma S, et al: Systematic review and meta-analysis of the clinical factors associated with the suicide of psychiatric in-patients. Acta Psychiatr Scand 124(1):18–29, 2011c 21261599

Lawrence D, Mitrou F, Zubrick SR: Smoking and mental illness: results from population surveys in Australia and the United States. BMC Public Health 9:285, 2009 19664203

Légaré F, Witteman HO: Shared decision making: examining key elements and barriers to adoption into routine clinical practice. Health Aff (Millwood) 32(2):276–284, 2013 23381520

Légaré F, Ratté S, Gravel K, Graham ID: Barriers and facilitators to implementing shared decision-making in clinical practice: update of a systematic review of health professionals' perceptions. Patient Educ Couns 73(3):526–535, 2008 18752915

Leikauf J, Schechter CB, Marrone K, et al: Patient-clinician agreement on treatment type and helpfulness: results from a WTC rescue and recovery worker cohort. Psychiatr Serv 64(11):1173–1176, 2013 24185541

Lemogne C, Nabi H, Melchior M, et al: Mortality associated with depression as compared with other severe mental disorders: a 20-year follow-up study of the GAZEL cohort. J Psychiatr Res 47(7):851–857, 2013 23590806

Leng JC, Changrani J, Tseng CH, Gany F: Detection of depression with different interpreting methods among Chinese and Latino primary care patients: a randomized controlled trial. J Immigr Minor Health 12(2):234–241, 2010 19408119

Lenzenweger MF, Lane MC, Loranger AW, Kessler RC: DSM-IV personality disorders in the National Comorbidity Survey Replication. Biol Psychiatry 62(6):553–564, 2007 17217923

Leucht S, Burkard T, Henderson J, et al: Physical illness and schizophrenia: a review of the literature. Acta Psychiatr Scand 116(5):317–333, 2007 17919153

Leykin Y, Derubeis RJ, Gallop R, et al: The relation of patients' treatment preferences to outcome in a randomized clinical trial. Behav Ther 38(3):209–217, 2007 17697846

Li Z, Page A, Martin G, Taylor R: Attributable risk of psychiatric and socio-economic factors for suicide from individual-level, population-based studies: a systematic review. Soc Sci Med 72(4):608–616, 2011 21211874

Lim RF (ed): Clinical Manual of Cultural Psychiatry, 2nd Edition. Washington, DC, American Psychiatric Publishing, 2015

Lin P, Campbell DG, Chaney EF, et al: The influence of patient preference on depression treatment in primary care. Ann Behav Med 30(2):164–173, 2005 16173913

Liu RT, Miller I: Life events and suicidal ideation and behavior: a systematic review. Clin Psychol Rev 34(3):181–192, 2014 24534642

Locatis C, Williamson D, Gould-Kabler C, et al: Comparing in-person, video, and telephonic medical interpretation. J Gen Intern Med 25(4):345–350, 2010 20107916

Lu W, Yanos PT, Silverstein SM, et al: Public mental health clients with severe mental illness and probable posttraumatic stress disorder: trauma exposure and correlates of symptom severity. J Trauma Stress 26(2):266–273, 2013 23508645

Makoul G, Clayman ML: An integrative model of shared decision making in medical encounters. Patient Educ Couns 60(3):301–312, 2006 16051459

Mamykina L, Vawdrey DK, Stetson PD, et al: Clinical documentation: composition or synthesis? J Am Med Inform Assoc 19(6):1025–1031, 2012 22813762

Mann JJ, Arango VA, Avenevoli S, et al: Candidate endophenotypes for genetic studies of suicidal behavior. Biol Psychiatry 65(7):556–563, 2009 19201395

Markkula N, Härkänen T, Perälä J, et al: Mortality in people with depressive, anxiety and alcohol use disorders in Finland. Br J Psychiatry 200(2):143–149, 2012 22157799

McGinty EE, Zhang Y, Guallar E, et al: Cancer incidence in a sample of Maryland residents with serious mental illness. Psychiatr Serv 63(7):714–717, 2012 22752037

McGinty EE, Baker SP, Steinwachs DM, Daumit G: Injury risk and severity in a sample of Maryland residents with serious mental illness. Inj Prev 19(1):32–37, 2013 22661205

McIntyre RS, Konarski JZ, Mancini DA, et al: Measuring the severity of depression and remission in primary care: validation of the HAMD-7 scale. CMAJ 173(11):1327–1334, 2005 16301700

Meeks TW, Wetherell JL, Irwin MR, et al: Complementary and alternative treatments for late-life depression, anxiety, and sleep disturbance: a review of randomized controlled trials. J Clin Psychiatry 68(10):1461–1471, 2007 17960959

Mergl R, Henkel V, Allgaier AK, et al: Are treatment preferences relevant in response to serotonergic antidepressants and cognitive-behavioral therapy in depressed primary care patients? Results from a randomized controlled trial including a patients' choice arm. Psychother Psychosom 80(1):39–47, 2011 20975325

Merinder LB, Viuff AG, Laugesen HD, et al: Patient and relative education in community psychiatry: a randomized controlled trial regarding its effectiveness. Soc Psychiatry Psychiatr Epidemiol 34(6):287–294, 1999 10422481 *

Mezzich JE, Caracci G, Fabrega H Jr, Kirmayer LJ: Cultural formulation guidelines. Transcult Psychiatry 46(3):383–405, 2009 19837778

Miller BJ, Paschall CB 3rd, Svendsen DP: Mortality and medical comorbidity among patients with serious mental illness. Psychiatr Serv 57(10):1482–1487, 2006 17035569

Milner A, Page A, LaMontagne AD: Long-term unemployment and suicide: a systematic review and meta-analysis. PLoS One 8(1):e51333, 2013 23341881

Miranda J, Duan N, Sherbourne C, et al: Improving care for minorities: can quality improvement interventions improve care and outcomes for depressed minorities? Results of a randomized, controlled trial. Health Serv Res 38(2):613–630, 2003 12785564

Mitchell AJ, Malone D, Doebbeling CC: Quality of medical care for people with and without comorbid mental illness and substance misuse: systematic review of comparative studies. Br J Psychiatry 194(6):491–499, 2009 19478286

Mitchell AJ, Lord O, Malone D: Differences in the prescribing of medication for physical disorders in individuals with v. without mental illness: meta-analysis. Br J Psychiatry 201(6):435–443, 2012 23209089

Mojtabai R, Olfson M: National trends in psychotropic medication polypharmacy in office-based psychiatry. Arch Gen Psychiatry 67(1):26–36, 2010 20048220

Morden NE, Lai Z, Goodrich DE, et al: Eight-year trends of cardiometabolic morbidity and mortality in patients with schizophrenia. Gen Hosp Psychiatry 34(4):368–379, 2012 22516216

Moriarty DG, Zack MM, Kobau R: The Centers for Disease Control and Prevention's Healthy Days Measures—population tracking of perceived physical and mental health over time. Health Qual Life Outcomes 1:37, 2003 14498988

Mościcki EK: Epidemiology of completed and attempted suicide: toward a framework for prevention. Clin Neurosci Res 1(5):310–323, 2001

Moulton B, King JS: Aligning ethics with medical decision-making: the quest for informed patient choice. J Law Med Ethics 38(1):85–97, 2010 20446987

Moye J, Sabatino CP, Weintraub Brendel R: Evaluation of the capacity to appoint a healthcare proxy. Am J Geriatr Psychiatry 21(4):326–336, 2013 23498379

Moyer VA; Preventive Services Task Force: Screening and behavioral counseling interventions in primary care to reduce alcohol misuse: U.S. preventive services task force recommendation statement. Ann Intern Med 159(3):210–218, 2013 23698791

Mueller TI, Leon AC, Keller MB, et al: Recurrence after recovery from major depressive disorder during 15 years of observational follow-up. Am J Psychiatry 156(7):1000–1006, 1999 10401442

Mueser KT, Goodman LB, Trumbetta SL, et al: Trauma and posttraumatic stress disorder in severe mental illness. J Consult Clin Psychol 66(3):493–499, 1998 9642887

Mundt JC, Clarke GN, Burroughs D, et al: Effectiveness of antidepressant pharmacotherapy: the impact of medication compliance and patient education. Depress Anxiety 13(1):1–10, 2001 11233454 *

Myers ED, Branthwaite A: Out-patient compliance with antidepressant medication. Br J Psychiatry 160:83–86, 1992 1544017 *

Narrow WE, Clarke DE, Kuramoto SJ, et al: DSM-5 field trials in the United States and Canada, Part III: development and reliability testing of a cross-cutting symptom assessment for DSM-5. Am J Psychiatry 170(1):71–82, 2013 23111499

National Commission for the Protection of Human Subjects of Biomedical and Behavioral Research: The Belmont Report: Ethical Principles and Guidelines for the Protection of Human Subjects of Research. Washington, DC, U.S. Government Printing Office, April 18, 1979

National Research Council: Crossing the Quality Chasm: A New Health System for the 21st Century. Washington, DC, The National Academies Press, 2001

Newcomer JW, Hennekens CH: Severe mental illness and risk of cardiovascular disease. JAMA 298(15):1794–1796, 2007 17940236

Nock MK, Borges G, Bromet EJ, et al: Suicide and suicidal behavior. Epidemiol Rev 30:133–154, 2008 18653727

O'Connor E, Gaynes BN, Burda BU, et al: Screening for and treatment of suicide risk relevant to primary care: a systematic review for the U.S. Preventive Services Task Force. Ann Intern Med 158(10):741–754, 2013 23609101

Olthuis G, Leget C, Grypdonck M: Why shared decision making is not good enough: lessons from patients. J Med Ethics 40(7):493–495, 2014 23660518

Oram S, Trevillion K, Feder G, Howard LM: Prevalence of experiences of domestic violence among psychiatric patients: systematic review. Br J Psychiatry 202:94–99, 2013 23377208

Osborn DP, Nazareth I, King MB: Risk for coronary heart disease in people with severe mental illness: cross-sectional comparative study in primary care. Br J Psychiatry 188:271–277, 2006 16507970

Osborn DP, Levy G, Nazareth I, et al: Relative risk of cardiovascular and cancer mortality in people with severe mental illness from the United Kingdom's General Practice Research Database. Arch Gen Psychiatry 64(2):242–249, 2007 17283292

Owen GS, Szmukler G, Richardson G, et al: Decision-making capacity for treatment in psychiatric and medical in-patients: cross-sectional, comparative study. Br J Psychiatry 203(6):461–467, 2013 23969482

Palmier-Claus JE, Ainsworth J, Machin M, et al: The feasibility and validity of ambulatory self-report of psychotic symptoms using a smartphone software application. BMC Psychiatry 12:172, 2012 23075387

Parks J, Svendsen D, Singer P, FotiME (eds); National Association of State Mental Health Program Directors (NAS MHPD) Medical Directors Council: Morbidity and mortality in people with serious mental illness. Alexandria, VA, National Association of State Mental Health Program Directors Medical Directors Council, October 2006

Patten SB, Williams JV, Lavorato DH, et al: Recall of recent and more remote depressive episodes in a prospective cohort study. Soc Psychiatry Psychiatr Epidemiol 47(5):691–696, 2012 21533819

Piatt EE, Munetz MR, Ritter C: An examination of premature mortality among decedents with serious mental illness and those in the general population. Psychiatr Serv 61(7):663–668, 2010 20592000

Pitschel-Walz G, Bäuml J, Bender W, et al: Psychoeducation and compliance in the treatment of schizophrenia: results of the Munich Psychosis Information Project Study. J Clin Psychiatry 67(3):443–452, 2006 16649832 *

Pokorny AD: Prediction of suicide in psychiatric patients: report of a prospective study. Arch Gen Psychiatry 40(3):249–257, 1983 6830404 *

Pokorny AD: Suicide prediction revisited. Suicide Life Threat Behav 23(1):1–10, 1993 8475527 *

Posner J, Eilenberg J, Friedman JH, Fullilove MJ: Quality and use of trauma histories obtained from psychiatric outpatients: a ten-year follow-up. Psychiatr Serv 59(3):318–321, 2008 18308915

Primm AB: Understanding the significance of race in the psychiatric clinical setting. FOCUS. The Journal of Lifelong Learning in Psychiatry 4(1):6–8, 2006

Procyshyn RM, Barr AM, Brickell T, Honer WG: Medication errors in psychiatry: a comprehensive review. CNS Drugs 24(7):595–609, 2010 20356315

Ravindran AV, da Silva TL: Complementary and alternative therapies as add-on to pharmacotherapy for mood and anxiety disorders: a systematic review. J Affect Disord 150(3):707–719, 2013 23769610

Redelmeier DA, Tu JV, Schull MJ, et al: Problems for clinical judgement, 2: obtaining a reliable past medical history. CMAJ 164(6):809–813, 2001 11276550

Rengarajan A, Mullins ME: How often do false-positive phencyclidine urine screens occur with use of common medications? Clin Toxicol (Phila) 51(6):493–496, 2013 23697457

Robinson GL, Gilbertson AD, Litwack L: The effects of a psychiatric patient education to medication program on post-discharge compliance. Psychiatr Q 58(2):113–118, 1986–1987 3562679 *

Robinson L, Dickinson C, Rousseau N, et al: A systematic review of the effectiveness of advance care planning interventions for people with cognitive impairment and dementia. Age Ageing 41(2):263–269, 2012 22156555

Rogers E, Sherman S: Tobacco use screening and treatment by outpatient psychiatrists before and after release of the American Psychiatric Association treatment guidelines for nicotine dependence. Am J Public Health 104(1):90–95, 2014 24228666

Rosenbloom ST, Denny JC, Xu H, et al: Data from clinical notes: a perspective on the tension between structure and flexible documentation. J Am Med Inform Assoc 18(2):181–186, 2011 21233086

Roshanaei-Moghaddam B, Katon W: Premature mortality from general medical illnesses among persons with bipolar disorder: a review. Psychiatr Serv 60(2):147–156, 2009 19176408

Rossegger A, Gerth J, Seewald K, et al: Current obstacles in replicating risk assessment findings: a systematic review of commonly used actuarial instruments. Behav Sci Law 31(1):154–164, 2013 23408438

Rush AJ, Gullion CM, Basco MR, et al: The Inventory of Depressive Symptomatology (IDS): psychometric properties. Psychol Med 26(3):477–486, 1996 8733206

Rush AJ Jr, First MB, Blacker D (eds): Handbook of Psychiatric Measures, 2nd Edition. Washington, DC, American Psychiatric Publishing, 2008

Ryan GJ, Caudle JM, Rhee MK, et al: Medication reconciliation: comparing a customized medication history form to a standard medication form in a specialty clinic (CAMPII 2). J Patient Saf 9(3):160–168, 2013 23965839

Saha S, Chant D, McGrath J: A systematic review of mortality in schizophrenia: is the differential mortality gap worsening over time? Arch Gen Psychiatry 64(10):1123–1131, 2007 17909124

Salsberry PJ, Chipps E, Kennedy C: Use of general medical services among Medicaid patients with severe and persistent mental illness. Psychiatr Serv 56(4):458–462, 2005 15812097

Sandson NB, Armstrong SC, Cozza KL: An overview of psychotropic drug-drug interactions. Psychosomatics 46(5):464–494, 2005 16145193

Saunders JB, Aasland OG, Babor TF, et al: Development of the Alcohol Use Disorders Identification Test (AUDIT): WHO collaborative project on early detection of persons with harmful alcohol consumption–II. Addiction 88(6):791–804, 1993 8329970

Schmidt CW, Yowell RK, Jaffe E: Procedure Coding Handbook for Psychiatrists, 4th Edition. Washington, DC, American Psychiatric Publishing, 2010

Selbæk G, Engedal K, Bergh S: The prevalence and course of neuropsychiatric symptoms in nursing home patients with dementia: a systematic review. J Am Med Dir Assoc 14(3):161–169, 2013 23168112

Sessums LL, Zembrzuska H, Jackson JL: Does this patient have medical decision-making capacity? JAMA 306(4):420–427, 2011 21791691

Sheridan SL, Harris RP, Woolf SH; Shared Decision-Making Workgroup of the U.S. Preventive Services Task Force: Shared decision making about screening and chemoprevention. a suggested approach from the U.S. Preventive Services Task Force. Am J Prev Med 26(1):56–66, 2004 14700714

Shiffman RN, Dixon J, Brandt C, et al: The GuideLine Implementability Appraisal (GLIA): development of an instrument to identify obstacles to guideline implementation. BMC Med Inform Decis Mak 5:23, 2005 16048653

Simon GE, Rutter CM, Stewart C, et al: Response to past depression treatments is not accurately recalled: comparison of structured recall and patient health questionnaire scores in medical records. J Clin Psychiatry 73(12):1503–1508, 2012 23290322

Sinclair LI, Davies SJC, Parton G, Potokar JP: Drug-drug interactions in general hospital and psychiatric hospital in-patients prescribed psychotropic medications. Int J Psychiatry Clin Pract 14(3):212–219, 2010 24917322

Singh JA, Sloan JA, Atherton PJ, et al: Preferred roles in treatment decision making among patients with cancer: a pooled analysis of studies using the Control Preferences Scale. Am J Manag Care 16(9):688–696, 2010 20873956

Singh JP, Fazel S, Gueorguieva R, Buchanan A: Rates of violence in patients classified as high risk by structured risk assessment instruments. Br J Psychiatry 204(3):180–187, 2014 24590974

Singh JP, Serper M, Reinharth J, Fazel S: Structured assessment of violence risk in schizophrenia and other psychiatric disorders: a systematic review of the validity, reliability, and item content of 10 available instruments. Schizophr Bull 37(5):899–912, 2011 21860036

Skevington SM, Lotfy M, O'Connell KA; WHOQOL Group: The World Health Organization's WHOQOL-BREF quality of life assessment: psychometric properties and results of the international field trial. A report from the WHOQOL group. Qual Life Res 13(2):299–310, 2004 15085902

Skinner HA: The drug abuse screening test. Addict Behav 7(4):363–371, 1982 7183189

Slade M, McCrone P, Kuipers E, et al: Use of standardised outcome measures in adult mental health services: randomised controlled trial. Br J Psychiatry 189:330–336, 2006 17012656

Smedley BD, Stith AY, Nelson AR (eds); Committee on Understanding and Eliminating Racial and Ethnic Disparities in Health Care: Unequal Treatment: Confronting Racial and Ethnic Disparities in Healthcare. Washington, DC, Institute of Medicine of the National Academies, 2003. Available at: http://www.nap.edu/openbook.php?record_id=12875&page=R1. Accessed September 14, 2012.

Smith SM, Stinson FS, Dawson DA, et al: Race/ethnic differences in the prevalence and co-occurrence of substance use disorders and independent mood and anxiety disorders: results from the National Epidemiologic Survey on Alcohol and Related Conditions. Psychol Med 36(7):987–998, 2006 16650344

Sobell LC, Brown J, Leo GI, Sobell MB: The reliability of the Alcohol Timeline Followback when administered by telephone and by computer. Drug Alcohol Depend 42(1):49–54, 1996 8889403

Soulier MF, Maislen A, Beck JC: Status of the psychiatric duty to protect, circa 2006. J Am Acad Psychiatry Law 38(4):457–473, 2010 21156904

Srebnik D, Appelbaum PS, Russo J: Assessing competence to complete psychiatric advance directives with the competence assessment tool for psychiatric advance directives. Compr Psychiatry 45(4):239–245, 2004 15224265

Stacey D, Bennett CL, Barry MJ, et al: Decision aids for people facing health treatment or screening decisions. Cochrane Database Syst Rev (10):CD001431, 2011 21975733

Stasiewicz PR, Vincent PC, Bradizza CM, et al: Factors affecting agreement between severely mentally ill alcohol abusers' and collaterals' reports of alcohol and other substance abuse. Psychol Addict Behav 22(1):78–87, 2008 18298233 *

Steidtmann D, Manber R, Arnow BA, et al: Patient treatment preference as a predictor of response and attrition in treatment for chronic depression. Depress Anxiety 29(10):896–905, 2012 22767424

Sterling RC, Gottheil E, Glassman SD, et al: Patient treatment choice and compliance: data from a substance abuse treatment program. Am J Addict 6(2):168–176, 1997 *

Sullivan JT, Sykora K, Schneiderman J, et al: Assessment of alcohol withdrawal: the revised clinical institute withdrawal assessment for alcohol scale (CIWA-Ar). Br J Addict 84(11):1353–1357, 1989 2597811

Sullivan JT, Fiellin DA, O'Connor PG: The prevalence and impact of alcohol problems in major depression: a systematic review. Am J Med 118(4):330–341, 2005 15808128

Swanson JW, Holzer CE 3rd, Ganju VK, Jono RT: Violence and psychiatric disorder in the community: evidence from the Epidemiologic Catchment Area surveys. Hosp Community Psychiatry 41(7):761–770, 1990 2142118

Swanson JW, Swartz MS, Van Dorn RA, et al; CATIE investigators: Comparison of antipsychotic medication effects on reducing violence in people with schizophrenia. Br J Psychiatry 193(1):37–43, 2008 18700216

Ten Have M, de Graaf R, van Weeghel J, van Dorsselaer S: The association between common mental disorders and violence: to what extent is it influenced by prior victimization, negative life events and low levels of social support? Psychol Med 44(7):1485–1498, 2014 24001369

The Joint Commission: Advancing Effective Communication, Cultural Competence, and Patient- and Family-Centered Care: A Roadmap for Hospitals. Oakbrook Terrace, IL, The Joint Commission, 2010. Available at: http://www.jointcommission.org/assets/1/6/ARoadmapforHospitalsfinalversion727.pdf. Accessed September 16, 2012.

The Joint Commission: Advancing Effective Communication, Cultural Competence, and Patient- and Family-Centered Care for the Lesbian, Gay, Bisexual, and Transgender (LGBT) Community: A Field Guide. Oakbrook Terrace, IL, The Joint Commission, October 2011. Available at: http://www.jointcommission.org/assets/1/18/LGBTFieldGuide.pdf. Accessed September 16, 2012.

The WHOQOL Group: Development of the World Health Organization WHOQOL-BREF quality of life assessment. Psychol Med 28(3):551–558, 1998 9626712

Thomas C, Kreisel SH, Oster P, et al: Diagnosing delirium in older hospitalized adults with dementia: adapting the Confusion Assessment Method to ICD-10 diagnostic criteria. J Am Geriatr Soc 60(8):1471–1477, 2012 22881707

Thomas M, Boggs AA, DiPaula B, Siddiqi S: Adverse drug reactions in hospitalized psychiatric patients. Ann Pharmacother 44(5):819–825, 2010 20371749

Thomas S, Leese M, Walsh E, et al: A comparison of statistical models in predicting violence in psychotic illness. Compr Psychiatry 46(4):296–303, 2005 16175762

Thomas SB, Quinn SC, Butler J, et al: Toward a fourth generation of disparities research to achieve health equity. Annu Rev Public Health 32:399–416, 2011 21219164

Thombs BD, Bennett W, Ziegelstein RC, et al: Cultural sensitivity in screening adults for a history of childhood abuse: evidence from a community sample. J Gen Intern Med 22(3):368–373, 2007 17356970

Tondora J, O'Connell M, Miller R, et al: A clinical trial of peer-based culturally responsive person-centered care for psychosis for African Americans and Latinos. Clin Trials 7(4):368–379, 2010 20571133

Toot S, Devine M, Akporobaro A, Orrell M: Causes of hospital admission for people with dementia: a systematic review and meta-analysis. J Am Med Dir Assoc 14(7):463–470, 2013 23510826

Trivedi MH: Tools and strategies for ongoing assessment of depression: a measurement-based approach to remission. J Clin Psychiatry 70(Suppl 6):26–31, 2009 19922741

Trivedi MH, Kern JK, Grannemann BD, et al: A computerized clinical decision support system as a means of implementing depression guidelines. Psychiatr Serv 55(8):879–885, 2004 15292537

Trivedi MH, Rush AJ, Gaynes BN, et al: Maximizing the adequacy of medication treatment in controlled trials and clinical practice: STAR(*)D measurement-based care. Neuropsychopharmacology 32(12):2479–2489, 2007 17406651

Tully MP, Ashcroft DM, Dornan T, et al: The causes of and factors associated with prescribing errors in hospital inpatients: a systematic review. Drug Saf 32(10):819–836, 2009 19722726

U.S. Census Bureau: American Community Survey 1-Year Estimates. Selected social characteristics in the United States, 2010; Available at: http://factfinder.census.gov/faces/tableservices/jsf/pages/productview.xhtml?pid=ACS_10_1YR_DP02&prodType=table. Accessed September 15, 2012.

U.S. Department of Health and Human Services: National standards for culturally and linguistically appropriate services in health and health care (the National CLAS Standards). Office of Minority Health, U.S. Department of Health and Human Services, 2013. Available at: http://minorityhealth.hhs.gov/omh/browse.aspx?lvl=2&lvlid=53. Accessed October 5, 2014.

U.S. Preventive Services Task Force: Counseling and interventions to prevent tobacco use and tobacco-caused disease in adults and pregnant women: U.S. Preventive Services Task Force reaffirmation recommendation statement. Ann Intern Med 150(8):551–555, 2009 19380855

Unützer J, Katon W, Callahan CM, et al; IMPACT Investigators. Improving Mood-Promoting Access to Collaborative Treatment: Collaborative care management of late-life depression in the primary care setting: a randomized controlled trial. JAMA 288(22):2836–2845, 2002 12472325

Valenstein M, Adler DA, Berlant J, et al: Implementing standardized assessments in clinical care: now's the time. Psychiatr Serv 60(10):1372–1375, 2009 19797378

van de Sande R, Nijman HL, Noorthoorn EO, et al: Aggression and seclusion on acute psychiatric wards: effect of short-term risk assessment. Br J Psychiatry 199(6):473–478, 2011 22016437 *

van den Boogaard M, Pickkers P, van der Hoeven H, et al: Implementation of a delirium assessment tool in the ICU can influence haloperidol use. Crit Care 13(4):R131, 2009 19664260 *

Van Dorn R, Volavka J, Johnson N: Mental disorder and violence: is there a relationship beyond substance use? Soc Psychiatry Psychiatr Epidemiol 47(3):487–503, 2012 21359532

van Eijk MM, van Marum RJ, Klijn IA, et al: Comparison of delirium assessment tools in a mixed intensive care unit. Crit Care Med 37(6):1881–1885, 2009 19384206 *

Van Orden KA, Witte TK, Cukrowicz KC, et al: The interpersonal theory of suicide. Psychol Rev 117(2):575–600, 2010 20438238

Vandereycken W, Vansteenkiste M: Let eating disorder patients decide: providing choice may reduce early drop-out from inpatient treatment. Eur Eat Disord Rev 17(3):177–183, 2009 19306300 *

Veerbeek MA, Voshaar RC, Pot AM: Clinicians' perspectives on a Web-based system for routine outcome monitoring in old-age psychiatry in the Netherlands. J Med Internet Res 14(3):e76, 2012 22647771

Vega WA, Rodriguez MA, Gruskin E: Health disparities in the Latino population. Epidemiol Rev 31:99–112, 2009 19713270

Velligan DI, Weiden PJ, Sajatovic M, et al: Assessment of adherence problems in patients with serious and persistent mental illness: recommendations from the Expert Consensus Guidelines. J Psychiatr Pract 16(1):34–45, 2010 20098229

Vespa J, Lewis JM, Kreider RM: America's Families and Living Arrangements: 2012. Current Population Reports P20-570. Washington, DC, U.S. Census Bureau, 2013

Vreeland B, Minsky S, Yanos PT, et al: Efficacy of the team solutions program for educating patients about illness management and treatment. Psychiatr Serv 57(6):822–828, 2006 16754759 *

Wesson DR, Ling W; WHO ASSIST Working Group: The Alcohol, Smoking and Substance Involvement Screening Test (ASSIST): development, reliability and feasibility. Addiction 97(9):1183–1194, 2002 12199834

Whittington R, Hockenhull JC, McGuire J, et al: A systematic review of risk assessment strategies for populations at high risk of engaging in violent behaviour: update 2002–8. Health Technol Assess 17(50):i–xiv, 1–128, 2013 24176100

Wilder CM, Elbogen EB, Moser LL, et al: Medication preferences and adherence among individuals with severe mental illness and psychiatric advance directives. Psychiatr Serv 61(4):380–385, 2010 20360277 *

Wilson E, Chen AH, Grumbach K, et al: Effects of limited English proficiency and physician language on health care comprehension. J Gen Intern Med 20(9):800–806, 2005 16117746

Witlox J, Eurelings LS, de Jonghe JF, et al: Delirium in elderly patients and the risk of postdischarge mortality, institutionalization, and dementia: a meta-analysis. JAMA 304(4):443–451, 2010 20664045

Witt K, van Dorn R, Fazel S: Risk factors for violence in psychosis: systematic review and meta-regression analysis of 110 studies. PLoS ONE 8(2):e55942, 2013 23418482

Woltmann EM, Whitley R: Shared decision making in public mental health care: perspectives from consumers living with severe mental illness. Psychiatr Rehabil J 34(1):29–36, 2010 20615842

World Health Organization: Measuring Health and Disability: Manual for WHO Disability Assessment Schedule (WHODAS 2.0). Geneva, World Health Organization, 2010

Yager J, Kunkle R, Fochtmann LJ, et al: Who's your expert? Use of an expert opinion survey to inform development of American Psychiatric Association practice guidelines. Acad Psychiatry 38(3):376–382, 2014 24493361

Yamada AM, Brekke JS: Addressing mental health disparities through clinical competence not just cultural competence: the need for assessment of sociocultural issues in the delivery of evidence-based psychosocial rehabilitation services. Clin Psychol Rev 28(8):1386–1399, 2008 18778881

Yeung AS, Jing Y, Brenneman SK, et al: Clinical Outcomes in Measurement-based Treatment (Comet): a trial of depression monitoring and feedback to primary care physicians. Depress Anxiety 29(10):865–873, 2012 22807244

Zimmerman M, McGlinchey JB: Depressed patients' acceptability of the use of self-administered scales to measure outcome in clinical practice. Ann Clin Psychiatry 20(3):125–129, 2008a 18633738

Zimmerman M, McGlinchey JB: Why don't psychiatrists use scales to measure outcome when treating depressed patients? J Clin Psychiatry 69(12):1916–1919, 2008b 19192467

Zimmerman M, Chelminski I, Young D, Dalrymple K: Using outcome measures to promote better outcomes. Clinical Neuropsychiatry: Journal of Treatment Evaluation 8:28–36, 2011

Zorina OI, Haueis P, Greil W, et al: Comparative performance of two drug interaction screening programmes analysing a cross-sectional prescription dataset of 84,625 psychiatric inpatients. Drug Saf 36(4):247–258, 2013 23494998

Zubkoff L, Young-Xu Y, Shiner B, et al: Usefulness of symptom feedback to providers in an integrated primary care--mental health care clinic. Psychiatr Serv 63(1):91–93, 2012 22227767

Disclosures

The Work Group on Psychiatric Evaluation and the Systematic Review Group reported the following conflicts of interest during development and approval of these guidelines, from May 2011 to December 2014:

Dr. Silverman is employed as a professor at Virginia Commonwealth University. He provides expert testimony to courts. He reports no conflicts of interest with his work on these guidelines.

Dr. Galanter is employed as a professor at the New York University Medical School. He reports no conflicts of interest with his work on these guidelines.

Dr. Jackson-Triche is employed as the chief mental health officer for the Sierra Pacific Network (VISN 21) of the U.S. Department of Veterans Affairs and as a professor at the University of California, Davis. She receives royalties from McGraw-Hill. She reports no conflicts of interest with her work on these guidelines.

Dr. Jacobs is a psychiatrist in private practice and on the faculty of Harvard Medical School, and provides medical-legal consultation, including expert testimony, on suicidality in psychiatric disorders, suicide causation, and related areas. He is the president of Screening for Mental Health and founder of National Depression Screening Day. He reports no conflicts of interest with his work on these guidelines.

Dr. Lomax is employed as a professor at Baylor College of Medicine. He reports no conflicts of interest with his work on these guidelines.

Dr. Riba is employed as a professor at the University of Michigan. She receives royalties from American Psychiatric Publishing, Saunders, Wiley, and Guilford. She reports no conflicts of interest with her work on these guidelines.

Dr. Tong is employed as a professor at the University of California, San Francisco. He receives royalty payments from Elsevier Publishing. He receives honoraria and travel funds from the National Board of Medical Examiners for test development. He reports no conflicts of interest with his work on these guidelines.

Dr. Watkins is employed as a researcher at the RAND Corporation and is a psychiatrist in private practice. She reports no conflicts of interest with her work on these guidelines.

Dr. Fochtmann is employed as a professor at Stony Brook University. She consults for the American Psychiatric Association on the development of practice guidelines. She has served as a stakeholder and as a technical expert panel member for AHRQ reviews related to psychiatric topics. She reports no conflicts of interest with her work on these guidelines.

Dr. Rhoads is employed an assistant professor at the University of Arizona and as a medical director for the University of Arizona Medical Center, South Campus, and the Crisis Response Center. He consults for the American Psychiatric Association on the development of practice guidelines. He reports no conflicts of interest with his work on these guidelines.

Dr. Yager is employed as a professor at the University of Colorado. He reports no conflicts of interest with his work on these guidelines.

Advisor to the Work Group

Michael J. Fitzpatrick, M.S.W.

Individuals and Organizations That Submitted Comments

Cesar Alfonso, M.D.
David M. Allen, M.D.
A.G. Awad, M.D.
Carl C. Bell, M.D.
B. Steven Bentsen, M.D., M.B.A.
Larry E. Beutler, Ph.D.
David Bloom, M.D.
Michael Blumenfield, M.D.
Jenny Boyer, M.D.
Robert C. Bransfield, M.D.
Rebecca Weintraub Brendel, M.D., J.D.
Lynn Bufka, Ph.D.
Ronald M. Burd, M.D.
Joseph R. Calabrese, M.D.
Linda L. Carpenter, M.D.
Catherine Chiles, M.D.
Mary Ann Adler Cohen, M.D.
Kate Comtois, Ph.D., M.P.H.
Catherine C. Crone, M.D.
Serina Deen, M.D., M.P.H.
Joel E. Dimsdale, M.D.
Nancy Donachie, M.D.
Jennifer I. Downey, M.D.
Farifteh Duffy, Ph.D.
R. Gregg Dwyer, M.D., Ed.D.
Denise M. Feil, M.D.
Marian Fireman, M.D.
Richard C. Friedman, M.D.
Keming Gao, M.D., Ph.D.
Sheila Hafter Gray, M.D.
Robert Greenberg, M.D.
Robert Gregory, M.D.
Elizabeth Haase, M.D.
Raquel Halfond, Ph.D.
Jill M. Harkavy-Friedman, Ph.D.
Tom W. Heinrich, M.D.
Gary M. Henschen, M.D.
Leon Hoffman, M.D.
Douglas H. Ingram, M.D.
Jeffrey S. Janofsky, M.D.
Margaret Jarvis, M.D.
Coni Kalinowski, M.D.
Kevin Kelly, M.D.
Lewis Kirshner, M.D.
Joseph C. Kobos, Ph.D.
David Koczerginski, M.D.
Thomas Kosten, M.D.
George Kowallis, M.D.
Harold Kudler, M.D.
Elisabeth Kunkel, M.D.

Molyn Leszcz, M.D.
Michael Marcangelo, M.D.
Eric R. Marcus, M.D.
John C. Markowitz, M.D.
William McDonald, M.D.
Samuel I. Miles, M.D.
Eve K. Mościcki, Sc.D., M.P.H.
Kim T. Mueser, Ph.D.
Juan C. Negrete, M.D.
Peter A. Olsson, M.D.
Narendra Patel, M.D.
Roger Peele, M.D.
Andrew T. Pickens, M.D.
Karen Pierce, M.D.
Ronald Pies, M.D.
Eric M. Plakun, M.D.
Seth Powsner, M.D.
Johanne Renaud, M.D., M.Sc.
John Rosenberger, M.D.
V. Sagar Sethi, M.D., Ph.D.
Peter A. Shapiro, M.D.
Michael Sharp, M.D.
Sanjeev Sockalingam, M.D.
Caroline Stamu-O'Brien, M.D.
David C. Steffens, M.D.
Jeffrey Sung, M.D.
Pamela J. Szeeley, M.D.
Ole J. Thienhaus, M.D.
Jeffrey Tuttle, M.D.
Kimerly A. Van Orden, Ph.D.
Erik R. Vanderlip, M.D.
Rajiv K. Vyas, M.D.
Stuart W.Twemlow, M.D.
John G. Wagnitz, M.D., M.S.
Elizabeth Weinberg, M.D.
Thomas N. Wise, M.D.
Linda L.M. Worley, M.D.

Academy of Psychosomatic Medicine
American Academy of Psychoanalysis and Dynamic
  Psychiatry
American Association for Marriage and Family Therapy
American Association for Geriatric Psychiatry
American Association for Social Psychiatry
American Group Psychotherapy Association
American Geriatrics Society
Magellan Health Services
Optum Behavioral Health
ValueOptions